CONCEPT OF HEALTH, HYGIENE AND MEDICINES

CONCEPT OF HEALTH, HYGIENE AND MEDICINES

A Study on Kondh Community of South Odisha

L.N. Raut
and
Bhabani Maharana

KALPAZ

ISBN : 978-93-5128-041-5

Published, 2018
Published by

Kalpaz Publications
C-30, Satyawati Nagar,
Delhi – 110052
www.gyanbooks.com
E-mail: kalpaz@hotmail.com
Ph.: 011-47034999, 9212142040

Printed at: G. Print Process, Delhi

Contents

Acknowledgements

It is a pleasant duty to acknowledge our indebtedness to a galaxy of persons who have helped us in different ways in the preparation of this work.

We are extremely grateful to the faculty members of the P.G. Department of History, Berhampur University for their help, support and cooperation.

We are highly indebted to Dr. Ananta Charan Sahoo, Ex-Director Academy of Tribal Language and Culture, Bhubaneswar and Former Deputy Director, Tribal Museum, SCSTRTI, Bhubaneswar who encouraged us at different levels for collection of required research data.

Our obligations are to Dr. Chitta Ranjan Satapathy for his cooperation and involvement in the preparation of this work.

Our heartiest thanks are also due to Dr. Balabhadra Tripathy for his inspiration and academic help to carry on this research work.

We are indebted to the authorities of different Libraries, Archives and Museums of Odisha State and outside for their help and cooperation in the collection of sources of materials. Our special thanks are due to the authorities of Central Library and

History SAP Library, Berhampur University for permitting us to utilise the source materials available with them freely.

L.N. Raut,

Bhabani Maharana

Introduction

Divided by the Tropic of Cancer and extending from the amazing altitudes of the Himalayas to the peninsular plateau dipping to the shores of vast Indian Ocean, India is the home to large number of tribal people, who are still untouched by the lifestyle of modern civilisation. Immensely vibrant and infinitely diverse, India, since time immemorial has been a rich treasure trove of tribal heritage. Complex and diverse culture, curious contrasts and phenomenal physical beauty are elements of intoxicating experience presented by tribal India. It is unique, perhaps unequalled in the richness and variety of its tribal life. Indian tribal people inhabit in approximately 15 per cent of the country's total area. They primarily reside in various ecological and geo-climatic conditions ranging from plains, forests, hills and inaccessible areas that perhaps, lie dotted in panoramic Indian terrain.

Lying on the eastern coast of India, kissing the sunlit waters of Bay of Bengal in the east and heavily forested blue hued hills of the Eastern Ghats, Odisha dazzles like a diamond with her elegance, refinement, grace, radiance, splendours, magnificence and rich tribal culture. Steeped in the mystery that surrounds their traditional habits and manners, the Odishan tribals continue to be a source of deep interest not only for anthropologists and social scientists but also for historians who flock to Odisha in search of the exotic mystique of this state. Odisha has the largest number of tribes, as many as 62, with a total population of 81, 45081 which constitutes an impressive 24 per cent of the state's total population. The state is a colourful canvas portraying a unique assimilation of various tribes, displaying varied culture and religion. The uniqueness lies in the fact that both ethnicity and culture go hand in hand and each influences the other. The diversity among the tribes is as kaleidoscopic as the non tribal population. Out of 62 tribes, 13 have been identified as primitive tribes in consideration of their pre-agricultural level of technology, low level of literacy and a stagnant or diminishing population.

The sixty two tribal communities that inhabit the state are widely different from one another in various ways. Each individual tribe is unique in terms of its material culture, settlement pattern, house type, mode of subsistence, social organisation, traditional decision making institutions, language, dance, music, adornment, food habit, tools and technologies, aesthetics, belief system, traditional practice of health and healing, use of forest medicinal plants and herbs for cure of diseases etc. The traditional and cultural distinction of each tribal community has made them distinguishable from each other. Their cultural and traditional heritages add colour and variation to the Indian culture as a whole and help to form a compact culture.

The tribals of Odisha reside in a contiguous belt. Almost all the districts of Odisha have tribal population. While some regions have huge presence and the other have handful of tribes. The districts cut by Eastern Ghats and Vindhyan ranges have a large percentage of tribal population. There are 15 major categories of tribes having a population of more then one lakh. They are: (i) Bhathudi, (ii) Bhottuda or Dhotada, (iii) Bhuyan, (iv) Bhumiji, (v) Gond, (vi) Kharia, (vii) Kandha or Kondh, (viii) Kissan, (ix) Kolha, (x) Munda, (xi) Oran, (xii) Paraja, (xiii) Santal, (xiv) Saora or Saura, and (xv) Lodha. The tribals of Odisha mainly inhabit in the districts of Mayurbhanj, Koraput, Malkangiri, Nowrangpur, Rayagada, Gajapati, Ganjam, Sundargarh, Keonjhar, Kandhamal and Kalahandi. These tribals, popularly known as *Adivasis* have always attracted the attention of anthropologists, sociologists and historians because they have remained more or less isolated from the rest of the world and have thus developed tendencies peculiar to their physique and social set up.

One of the largest tribal populations of the world lives in India. But in the Indian context 'tribe' has never been defined precisely and satisfactorily. It was used, at one time, to denote bewildering variety of social categories that were neither analogous nor comparable. The International Labour Organisation has classified such people as indigenous. The term *adivasi, girijan, vanyajati* and so on are of recent origin. Tribe is defined as a group of family which has common names, whose members speak a common dialect, reside in a common area, observe taboo in marriage and occupation, have a common interest and have a well developed reciprocal exchange. They are distinguished in terms of their territory, language, culture and tradition and development of reciprocity and mutuality of obligation. Like the other societies, the tribal society is also not static rather it is quite dynamic. The rate of change in this society is very slow. That is why they have been underdeveloped and poor compared to other people. The English term 'tribe' comes from the Latin word *tribus*, designating a particular kind of social and political organisation existing in all these societies. The term refers to the largest kind of social and political community with internal sub-division or segments and there is an internal relationship real or implied between kinship and political organisation.

The tribals are the indigenous inhabitants of India. They constitute a disadvantaged sector of the Indian society. Their political awareness is very low because of their poverty, illiteracy and social backwardness. They have been living in different parts of the country before the Aryans penetrated into India. They slowly but certainly, obliged them by moving bit by bit into the interior areas. The tribals have lived far away from the mainstream for centuries, in the relatively isolated, inaccessible, less fertile and less agriculturally productive region of forests, hills and mountains. They have been denied the basic human rights. They have also been subjected to social injustice and economic exploitation for centuries. They have been reeling under the tyranny of the *Zamindars*, landlords, contractors, money lenders and other agencies and consequently remained at their mercy. On the other hand nature has taught them to love, respect and fear and worship forces of nature. The tribal societies share some common characteristics, which make them distinctly different from advanced and complex societies.

Among the *adivasis* or the schedule tribes, the Kondhs or the Kui as they called themselves are the most numerous. They have a great cultural heritage and values which respect nature. Customarily they were once notorious for their brutal acts of human sacrifice (*meriah*) to achieve the end products of bumper crops and for better yield of turmeric. There are various sections among Kondhs. Each section is endogamous though originally they hail from the same Kondh community. They express their cultural identity and distinctiveness in their social organisation, languages, rites and rituals, festivals including their dresses, ornaments, arts and crafts, food and drinking habits. Every facet of their life is intimately connected with religious beliefs, ritualistic practices and beliefs in supernatural powers. The geographical situation of the Kondh villages surrounded by hills and forests, away from the main developed areas and lacking in communication facilities stand in the way of a systematic improvement of health and hygienic conditions of the community. They have deep faith in the efficacy of divine blessing and magic of 'spirits' for cure with a strong belief that due to wrath of spirits one suffers from disease or disability. An isolated community away from the mainstream of civilisation lacks medical facilities curative as well as preventive. The Christian missionaries in isolated pockets extend medical help to the needy and facilities provided by Government are too meager. The Kondhs live in unhealthy and unhygienic condition. They do not get pure drinking water. One's earning is directly linked with one's diet. Average land holding is very little and avenues of employment are too limited. As the purchasing power of Kondh families being less, they are unable to procure minimum food. Besides this, protein content in their food is insignificant as they occasionally get protein from jungle or domestic animals and they are unable to supplement their diet with milk or pulses. The male members (to some extent females also) of the Kondh community are addicted to alcohol which creates repulsion and irregularity of food habits causing damage to the body system. Due to lack of awareness about health and hygiene the Kondhs suffer from a number of diseases. They suffer from malnutrition, malaria and anemia. Health services are insufficient and Kondh religious beliefs interfere with acceptance of modern medicine and healthy lifestyles. They use local herbs and medicinal plants to cure their illness. As a fish can not live without water, Kondhs can not live without forests. It is the source of their food, medicinal plants, and home to their god. The herbal medicines occupy a very important role in their indigenous methods of treatment which helps these people to get relieved of their mental and physical disorders.

Review of Literature

Although the Kondh culture and civilisation is very old, no comprehensive study about their health and hygiene has been made so far. Many works have been carried out on the socio-cultural, religious and economic life of Kondh people. A lot of works have been done on their evil practices which were going on among them since long back. But no serious attempt has been made so far to study about their health, hygiene and medicine, which constitute a major part of their life. The districts gazetteers and manuals like *Koraput District Gazeteer, Kandhamal District Gazeteer, Angul District Gazeteer, Ganjam District Manual* do not provide adequate information about this aspect of their life. These sources are totally insufficient to study the health, hygiene and medicinal practices of Kondh community. The records of missionaries about tribal Odisha also do not provide sufficient information about this vital aspect. The books which have been published so far do not endeavor to present the tribal beliefs, practices and their living condition, which has a great impact on their health. Some books have been published regarding the use of ethno-botany by this tribe for the cure of a number of diseases but they have not touched their living condition and mental state of this tribe which affect their health to a great extent.

There are few published memoirs by early British officers viz. Captain Samuel Charter Macpherson, Colonel John Campbell, R.V. Russel and V. Elwin who worked with the tribals and provide us with some information about the aboriginal tribes and their institutions. A few published articles are also available on the subject. Still a comprehensive historical study about health, hygiene and medicinal practices of Kondh community has not been done so far.

Objective of the Present Study

The main purport of this work is to present an in-depth, comprehensive and critical study about the concept of health, hygiene and medicine among the Kondhs of south Odisha, keeping in view the history and culture of the region. This humble effort aims at presenting a detailed, dispassionate and an analytical study on an important aspect of life and culture of this primitive people. Here a sincere attempt has been made to study the use of herbal medicine by this community and its importance for them. In spite of medical facilities still they prefer the plant as their first choice of medicine. They know the best use of each and every plant for their small requirements of day to day life.

Sources and Methodology

The work is mainly based on primary and secondary data available on the subject. Field visit has also been undertaken to gather first hand information on the subject. Plenty of records and references used in the preparation of this work have been taken from different institutions like Tamil Nadu State Archives, Chennai, Odisha State Archives, Bhubaneswar, Record Rooms of Board of Revenue, Cuttack, Collectorate of Ganjam, Koraput, Kandhamal, Angul and Vizagpatnum. *Gazeteers* published by the authority of the British Government and Government of Odisha also form a part of our source materials. Research data preserved in Odisha State Library, Odisha Assembly Library, Tribal Research Bureau Library, Parija Library (Utkal University), Scheduled Castes and Scheduled Tribes Research and Training Institute Library, Bhubaneswar; Council of Analytical Tribal Studies Library, Koraput, Kanika Library, Ravenshaw University, Cuttack; Special Assistance Programme Library, Seminar Library of History Department, Library of the Museum and Archival Cell, Central Libray of Berhampur University, Berhampur and M.S. Swaminathan Research Foundation, Library, Jeypore have been extensively used.

Area of Study

The area of study is limited to southern part of Odisha, comprising the districts of Ganjam, Gajapati, Koraput, Rayagada, Nabarangapur, Malkangiri, Boudh and Kandhamal. Though Kondh population is seen in a number of districts of Odisha, they inhabit in large numbers in these districts of south Odisha. These south Odishan districts are homeland to three major groups of Kondh community viz. Desia Kondhs, Kutia Kondhs and Dongaria Kondhs. That is why these regions of south Odisha have been chosen as area of study.

Chapterisation

The present work is structured into five chapters besides introduction and conclusion.

Chapter one presents a historical background, origin, area of habitation as well as place of Kondhs in the tribal community of Odisha. Attempt is also made to throw light on the climatic condition, flora and fauna of the area where the Kondhs live. This chapter also deals in detail about the different groups of Kondh community.

Chapter two deals with the concept of health and hygiene of this tribal community. Here a humble attempt has been made to discuss about the general health condition of Kondh people, their hygienic awareness and factors responsible for the degradation of their health standards. In this chapter study is also undertaken to highlight the environment, habitation and food habits of the Kondhs, which affect their health and living conditions in different ways.

Chapter three depicts the socio-religious practices of Kondh community. Their religious beliefs relating to health and diseases are discussed in detail. Their different gods and goddesses, role of *jani* and *disaries* in their socio-religious life are also highlighted. Attempt is also made to elaborate the taboos and some festivals celebrated by these people for the cure of some diseases and remedy to these maladies.

Chapter four aims at throwing light on use of various medicinal plants by the Kondhs for the cure of different diseases. Here an attempt is made to present different diseases, their local names, symptoms, the techniques of preparing herbal medicines and their application. The botanical names of the plants and roots are also mentioned.

Chapter five presents a comparative study of tribal medicine and modern medicine. The importance of traditional tribal medicine which survived till date with certain modifications is delineated herein.

The findings of the study are presented in the conclusion followed by bibliography, appendices and photographs with illustrations.

1

Kondh Community in Odisha

Odisha, one of the most picturesque and captivating states of India, nestling on the shore of Bay of Bengal is a land of unmatched beauty and amazing diversity. Washed by the waters of Bay of Bengal in the eastern coast, Odisha has the distinction of being endowed liberally with the bounties of nature.[1] Its extensive palm fringed coast line, serene holiday beaches, pronounced rural environment, charming blue hills rising here and there, green wood lands, rough caves, majestically roaming wild animals, exotic birds, fascinating sculptured temples, mud villages set in greens, modern industrial leviathans and colourful tribes make Odisha a miniature India. Here is *Bharat* in capsule. The footage of its cultural panorama is evidently witnessed in its sloppy mountains, sparkling spring, inky sky and dazzling plateau. It is a state embellished with a beautiful stretch of Indo-Aryan coast where modern life persists and hilly terrain of Eastern Ghats where primitive tribes dwell. Odisha has always taken an important, distinct and colourful position on the national map by harbouring various culturally unique ethnic tribal communities since time immemorial.

Odisha's bills and dales tell stories. Its trees and creepers sing and its people dance to the tune of music. This seems true when one visits the zoo of its ethnological groups of aborigine primitive people, who are emotional in nature and creative in spirit. The various tribes inhabiting the state present another spectrum of our civilisation. Their innocence, their love for culture and nature, their beliefs and practices, their art and artefacts provide a striking contrast to the ways of modern world.

Odisha, an integral part of Indian union is located in the eastern part of India extended between the parallels of 17°49′ North to 22°34′ North latitude and from 81°29′ East to 87°29′ East longitude. It is bounded by West Bengal in the north-east, Bihar in the north, Chhatisgarh in the west, Andhra Pradesh in the south and Bay of Bengal in the east. The state has an area of about 155,707 sq. km with a coastline of 482 km. It is basically a riverine state since many rivers big and small flow through the state to the Bay of Bengal.[2]

An important demographic feature of the state lies with the fact that its component of weaker section comprising scheduled castes and scheduled tribes claim two-fifth of the total population. The scheduled tribe people are roughly rounded off to 85 *lakhs* which is about 23.12 per cent of the total population. It is home to 62 distinct tribes including some of the most primitive tribes, each one with its own culture and traditions different from the other. Mostly of Proto-Australoid stock, many of the Odishan tribes are high land tribes with rich ethnological character and customs, varying language and dialects. The different tribes have long been able to reject the main land influence and have preserved their social customs, living style and technological values. In spite of the inroads of so called modern civilisation and developmental programmes, Odishan *adivasis* still lead a simple, traditional and colourful life. Tribal society displays a fascinating profile of ethnic diversity. The variation in physical and biological environment of their habitat is equally amazing. The bewildering variety in race, language, habitat and economy is fully reflected in their culture and living style.

Scholars have used the term 'tribe' to denote several social groups or communities who are culturally and linguistically homogeneous. The term is further associated with many useful connotations. Usually tribe and tribalism has been used by the British imperial historiographers. The term tribe is synonymous with aborigines and indigenous/local people. Whatever the variations may be for convenience, the use of term better is restricted to a specific group of Indian society. Original or native inhabitants of a country are otherwise known as indigenous people. The aborigines in Indian language are known as *adivasis*. These human groups are known as scheduled tribes or *anusuchita jati, vanjati, pahari, adimjati, vanabasi* etc.[3]

In order to understand the problem of variation among most of the tribes of Odisha, we first observe that an individual tribe has its hill dwelling division which is relatively different from the plains dwelling or foothill dwelling or plateau dwelling division. This dualism in habitation is important for an understanding of social, cultural and linguistic variations. Similarly, geographic location, physiographic condition of living, degree of isolation and exposure to the outer society are other factors important for understanding variations among tribes.[4]

Linguistically the tribes of India are broadly classified into four categories, viz. (i) Indo-Aryan speakers, (ii) Dravidian speakers, (iii) Tibeto-Burmese speakers and (iv) Austric speakers. In Odisha the speakers of the Tibeto-Burmese language family are absent, and therefore Odishan tribes belong to other three language families. The Indo-Aryan language family in Odisha includes Dhelki-Odia, Matia, Haleba, Jharia, Saunti, Laria and Odia (spoken by Bathudi and the acculturated sections of Bhuyan, Juang, Kondh, Savara, Raj Gond etc.). The Austric language family includes eighteen tribal languages namely, Birija, Perenga, Kisan, Bhumiju, Koda, Mahili, Bhumiji, Mirdha-Kharia, Ollar Gadaba, Juang, Bondo, Didayee, Karmali, Kharia, Munda, Ho, Mundari and Savara. Within the Dravidian language family there are nine languages in Odisha, viz. Pengo, Gondi, Kisan, Konda, Koya, Parji, Kui, Kuvi and Kurukh or Oraon.

Considering the general features of their eco system, traditional economy, supernatural beliefs and practices and recent “impact of modernisation”, the tribes of Odisha can be classified into six types, such as: (i) haunting, collecting and gathering type, (ii) cattle-herder type, (iii) simple artisan type, (iv) hill and shifting cultivation type, (v) settled agriculture type and (vi) industrial urban worker type.

From racial point of view the tribes can be broadly divided into three groups, viz. (i) Negritoes, (ii) Austroloid and (iii) Mongoloids. Most of the tribal communities living in the northern and north-eastern areas are of Mongoloid stock. The largest group of tribal community in India belongs to the Austroloid section. The tribal community of southern India has Negrito trait.[5]

Among all other tribes of Odisha, Kondh is one of the most colourful, real and primitive tribe living in the inaccessible dense forests and hilly terrains. They practise hill and shifting cultivation. In addition to this, their economy is also supported by haunting and fishing. They have racial affinity with proto-Austroloid stock. But some of the scholars have considered them proto-Austroloid mixed with Mongoloid elements. Proto-Austroloid and Mongoloid skeletons have been discovered from Harappa and Mohenjodaro remains. It can be therefore presumed that the distant forefathers of the Kondhs belonged to Indus Valley Civilisation. Consequent upon the gradual decline of the Indus Valley Civilisation the inhabitants marched towards the Gangetic valley and gradually to western and southern India and the Kondhs were no exception to this. It is also assumed that they also lived in the foot of Himalayas.[6] It is believed that Kondhs, who belonged to the non-Aryan section, settled on the foot of the Himalayas and gradually migrated in two parts. One group proceeded eastward and the other to the south up to the Vindhyas. The Vindhyan group first entered into the Kalahandi area of Odisha. Thereafter they were further divided into two groups. One group moved southward through Koraput district up to modern Andhra Pradesh region and the other group moved northwards to Bolangir, Sambalpur, Boudh and Kandhamala. On the basis of archaeological evidences, it seems that Kondhs settled in the Boudh-Kandhamala district and north-western region of the Ganjam district which adjoins the Kandhamala.[7] The British officers like R.V. Russell, Captain Samuel Charter Macpherson and John Campbell came to know about the community as early as the middle of the 19th century when they were deputed to the Kondh country for the suppression of the *meriah* prevalent in the Kondh society. The accounts given by these officers serve as the valuable source of information regarding the life style and culture of these people. They provide us with some data about their origin and place of settlement. There is no proper record so far as the derivation of the term Kondh and the origin of this tribe is concerned. There are different opinions of different scholars and deputed officers.[8]

According to Macpherson the term Kondh connects with Tamil word *Kandha* meaning thereby the inhabitant of the hills. Dalton holds the similar view. But Risley does not agree to it.[9] In Telugu language the Kondhs are called *Kodu vandulu*, in Odia *Kandha loka* and the *Kandha* call themselves *Kui* which is *Kuinga* in plural form. The name Kondh as Macpherson has suggested is derived from the Telugu word *Konda*, a hill as well as hill men. The territory in which the Kandha reside in large number is called the Kandhamala. *Mala* in Odia signifies a hill tract and the northern portion of the Ganjam district which adjoins Kandhamal is called the Kondh *Maliah* meaning the hill tracts inhabited by the Kondhs. This tribe is variously known as the Kond, Kondh or Kandha.[10] In course of time they have formed themselves into separate endogamous units and have developed considerable cultural and economic diversity.

Scholars have also tried to identify it with the Odia word *Khanda* which denotes to a piece of land accommodating a specific quantity of seeds to be shown. But this view is not acceptable. There is another theory. The word *Kandha* and *Skandha* means shoulder in Sanskrit. The Kondhs used to carry loads of wood on their shoulders which is the principal limb of the body. From the word *skandha* the word Kondh is derived. Another theory is given in this context in the *Ramayana*. It has been described that a tribe of *Asuras* called Skandasuras, who were known to have ruled over the hills and forest of Dandaka extending from Vindhyan hills to the river Krishna and the Kondhs may be a remnant of this tribe. The Kondhs as a whole are militant and as such they used to have always a sword in their hands. The sword in Odia language is *Khanda*. Hence, these people were called Kandha people. Subsequently from it the word Kondh has been derived. So without proper data nothing can be said about the origin of the name Kondh. Macpherson's opinion is more acceptable. The derivation of the name Kondh from Telugu word *Konda,* a hill, appears to be more plausible. This has been supported by Stephen Hislop.[11]

The legendary account of the origin of Kondhs reveals that once upon a time the ground was all wet and there were only two females on the earth named *Karaboodi* and *Tharthaboodi*, each of them blessed with a single male child. Those two children were *Kasarodi* and *Singarodi.* All these individuals sprang from the interior of the earth. Along with them two small plants called *Rangokoocha* and *Badokoocha* sprang up and on those plants they depended for their subsistence. Subsequently the wet soil dried up and from it all kinds of animals and trees came into existence. *Kosarodi* and *Singarodi* were given in marriage to the two daughters of *Bora Penu.* Kondhs believe that they have been originated from them as their children.

Macpherson has given another theory regarding the origin of the Kondhs. He writes, "no mythology and legend appears to exist amongst the Kondhs, which indicates, however dimly, their origin or from whence they are derived; they believe themselves to have existed in Odisha from the beginning, having either sprung from the soil itself like the branches of Greeks or having been created contemporaneously along with it." This hypothesis of Macpherson is corroborated by J.P. Frye.

A few other scholars have advanced another view. The earliest inhabitants of India were the Proto- Austroloids in whom there might be some infilteration of African or even Negrito blood in the coastal part of India at later periods. The Kondhs can be put to this Proto-Austroloid racial stock and might not be an independent race or otherwise. Some other scholars opine that the very earliest inhabitants of India are Negritos of the Andaman Island type. The earliest inhabitants have been depicted as a dark Negroid race that subsequently came in contact with the immigrants of higher culture possibly through Baluchistan. They established themselves in the north possibly between 4000 B.C. to 2500 B.C. and then spread over the Deccan in the south. Intercommunity marriage might have occurred between them. So it is presumed that the primitive existing race of India is the pre-Dravidians and the Kondhs belonged to this pre-Dravidian group.

It has been revealed from the earliest Aryan legends that the Aryans entered India between 1700 B.C. and 1300 B.C. and settled in the Indo-Gangetic basin. They were stronger in physique and large in numbers, hence succeeded in imposing their will on the weaker groups. They also compelled these weaker people either to surrender or to escape to the inaccessible areas of the forests and the mountains. The Kondhs belonged to these weaker groups. But these Kondhs in varying degrees have preserved their independence in these hills and since then they have been living independently. There is no reliable source to prove it and it is difficult to say whether the Kondhs were the original settlers of the low lands near to their present habitat or had migrated from the other region of our country.[12]

The old men of the community recall a mythical story that one *Sapangada* was the creator of this world. He created seven brothers. These brothers lived in a village called Gumma in Baliguda subdivision of Phulbani District. Seven deities namely *Raniadu, Bendiad, Pusharini, Deusadu, Tumbasadu, Udungdle* and *Betangdali* were created for seven brothers. These brothers were asked to satisfy the deities. Two out of the seven brothers who satisfied the deities became Odias. They were asked to eat goat only. Three other brothers could not satisfy the deities, therefore they became Kondhs. They were asked to eat buffalo. The remaining two brothers satisfied the deities half heartedly became *Panos* or *Dombs*. They were asked to eat cows. Thus the Kondh came to be known as *adi manab* (early man) from whom the *Panos* and Odias descended. In course of time the three brothers quarrelled with each other being cursed by *Sapangada* as they could not satisfy the deities. One of them hid himself in a *Kuti* (cave) and became untraceable. He was therefore known as Kutia Kondh. The second brother flew from the place and remained over a hill and became Dongria Kondh, whereas the third brother came to a river and took shelter under trees in a grove. He was known as Desia Kondh. In fact, the Kutias are considered to be the original Kondhs with their habitat in Gumma area of Kondhamala district where the cult of *Sapangada* still exists. Whatever may be the fact there are no records to prove the story as true and also to prove that other sections of the Kondhs are offshoots of the original Kutia Kondh.[13]

Kondhs of different places used to relate different stories of their origin. In the Kandhamala, the old men of the tribe maintain that in the days of yore they lived at a place called Srambuli Dimbuli adjoining the high range of hills named Derhsaru somewhere in Ganjam or the Central Provinces. When they were pushed back from the fertile lands below, they climbed the hills with courage and felt that they were at the end of the world. Meanwhile, they saw at a great distance a large tract of jungles apparently uninhabited. Hence they made up their minds to occupy the same. Then they promptly climbed the hills and took possession of the Kondhmala and the surrounding tracts. They found a few occupants there and they were soon ousted. They are now found in scattered hamlets of Daspalla and other neighbouring regions. But none except the Kondhs is to be seen within the Kondhmala. The people who were ousted are known as the *Kurmus* or *Kermis* living on cultivation and other peaceful employment. It is said that it was from them that the Kondhs learned the art of living on cultivation and other peaceful employments.

Freiend Pereira refers to another tradition that the Kondhs were driven away by a stronger race from the tract corresponding to the modern Gaya district and gradually found their way through Chhotnagpur and the Gondwana to the hills which form their present home.[14]

In 261 B.C. Ashoka conquered the kingdom of Kalinga (the ancient name of Odisha). During the war some tribals were known to have fled to the hill tracts. The Kondhs might be one of such tribes. Ashoka was kind to them. This has been reflected in the Rock Edict XIII. Kondhs had little contact with Aryans of the plain till the end of the third century A.D. It was in the fourth century A.D. during Gupta age that the Kondhs were known to have appeared in the political scenario of India.[15] Verrier Elwin was the first anthropologist in the country to give his impression about the tribe in the year 1943. Niggemeyar had published detailed ethnographic account of the Kutia Kondh in the year 1964. As it was written in German language many scholars do not have access to it.[16]

This tribe is variously known. They have considerable cultural diversity. *Kui* is their language but it has local variations. The Kondhs of Koraput sub-division speak *Kuvi* (or Kui) language. Kondhs of Baliguda sub division speak the *Kui* language. Kondhs of Gudari area speak *Kutia* which is a mixture of *Saura* and *Kui* dialects. Kondhs of Rayagada sub-division speak *Kuvi* mixed with Telugu. *Kuvi* appears to have original structural composition while *Kui* an acculturated and transformed form of *Kuvi* language. Many of the Kondhs have lost their mother tongue and speak Odia. Some have become bilingual because they speak Odia in the interior areas of the state and Telugu in border areas.[17] Kondhs are variously divided and thus not uniform in their structure or habit. Kondhs have two main divisions namely hill Kondhs and plain Kondhs. Hill Kondhs who reside in the hills have retained their primitive customs. The plain Kondhs dwelling in plain areas have acquired a tincture of Hinduism. H.H. Risley had named these two divisions as *Malua* or *Arria* Kondh and Oriya Kondh. Macpherson has divided the Kondhs into three principal classes namely *Benniah* Kondh, *Bethiah* Kondh and *Malliah* Kondh. Kondhs are again found with different names such as *Budha* Kondh, *Nanguli* Kondh, *Sita* Kondh, *Malua* Kondh, *Pengo* Kondh, *Muli* Kondh, *Jatapu* Kondh and *Kacharia* Kondh. *Kacharia* Kondhs are found in Kalahandi district. Kondhs inhabited in Kerandimala or Mohiri hill of Ganjam are called *Tinki* Kondhs. There is another group called *Raj* Kondh who considered themselves superior to all other sections. Hence they marry among themselves.[18] Kondhs are known by different names after their place of habitation, life style and culture. They are physically well built and remarkably active. According to the modern scholar Krishan Sharma the complexion of the Kondhs varies from light brown to brown. Their hair has a tendency to be rather wavy. The colour of their hair is dark brown and not very profuse in quantity. The beard and moustache in males are scanty. Their eyes are mostly dark brown with the iris red, the sclera predominantly yellow, dull and speckled. Their eye slits vary from straight to oblique. In some the presence of the eye fold is visible. Eyebrows are medium and separate. Lips are of medium thickness. Nasal indexes vary from peatyrrline to mesorrline. The nasal profile is predominantly concave. The incisor folds are marked and the body is generally athletic.[19]

Kondh women are diminutive in stature and coarse in features. They have habit of tattooing their faces and smearing themselves with turmeric.[20] Kondhs are well accustomed to jungle life. They are cheerful, mobile, reserved, self possessed, generous and polite, glad to talk with one who knows their language. They are bold, laborious and upright in their conduct. Kondhs are faithful to their friends. They are simple minded enough to prefer a truth to a lie. The kondhs are great lovers of liberty. Intellectually, they are also by no means dull and stupid. Every stranger is an invited guest. As soon as a traveller enters in a village, the heads of the families respectfully solicit him to share their meal. He may remain as long as he desires. A guest can never be turned away. Fugitives from the field of battle and even escaped criminals must be hospitably received. Thus the Kondhs treat any stranger of any rank, as an equal.[21] However, there are some vices in the character of the Kondhs. Some anthropologists and British officials have also discovered such vices in them. H.H. Risley depicts the Kondhs as shy, timid and hate to have contact with the inhabitants of the plains. Verrier Elwin also described them as most difficult, timid and suspicious of all the Orissan high landers. Perhaps he has stated this due to their long conflict with government over human sacrifice and infanticide.[22] Colonel Campbell writes, "Kondhs sunk in the depths of ignorance, superstition and sensuality." They are not so expert at a lie as their more civilised neighbours of the plains but regard for truth for its own sake they have none. But his description seems to be one sided. That is because he never lived amongst the Kondhs. He only marched through the country in the winter months in order to suppress human sacrifice.

Of course it is true that the Kondhs are very superstitious, ignorant and addicted to drink. Occasionally they show their love of revenge and even for brutal passion.[23] G.F. Paddison has made a special study of Kondh's problem in 1916 and submitted a report to the Madras Government. In his report he has mentioned that by that time Kondhs had lost many of the good qualities in their character and that was largely due to their intercourse with the people of the plains.[24] Although Kondhs are of different categories but broadly they are divided into three groups depending upon their habitat such as *Kutia, Dongria* and *Desia*.

The Kutia (hill) Kondh is the weakest section leading an isolated life of poverty and indigence. The Dongria (hill) Kondh is comparatively less primitive and more skilled in horticulture. The Desia (low country) Kondhs have left their hill and settled down in plains to pursue cultivation.[25]

The Kondhs are different to each other as per their choice of food, living style and beliefs. They consider themselves as the original inhabitants of the soil. According to them "this is our soil, the earth is our mother and we always appease her by regular worshipping because she provides us food".[26] This shows their innocence and patriotic feeling. They love their motherland more than their life. They identify themselves as *Kui, Kuinga, Kui Enju, Kui loka or Kui lok,* etc., but their neighbours call them Kondh.[27] Living in an inhospitable terrain, in the wild and hilly areas, being isolated from the more civilised people of the plains and largely unaware of rapid changes there, the Kondhs have preserved the primitive system of social organisation. They furnish an interesting example of a primitive race of improvident social customs and habits.

Kutia Kondh

Kutia Kondh is one of the most primitive sub-tribes of the Kondh tribe. The term Kutia means "big hole in earth". They relate closely to the Proto-Austroloid stock with considerable Mongoloid admixture. They live in small settlements on the slopes of the hills. They are found in Belghar, Gumma, Lankagarh, Jharipani *Gram Panchayat* in Tumudibandh block and few villages of Subarnagiri area of Kotagarh block in Kandhamala district. This sub-tribe is also found in Lanjigarh block of Kalahandi District. Kutia generally called *Kuinga* means "above or top of hill" and they speak *Kui* language. The Kondh in general and the Kutia in particular display a character of normal conduct.

From the origin and course of development of settlement it is ascertained that Kutia Kondh villages were uniclan. But gradually most of the villages are now found to be inhabited by multiclan groups and people of other ethnic groups. However, strong feeling of community co-operation, as the basic characteristic feature of Kutia Kondh settlement, so far exists.

While selecting a site for habitation, the traditional magico-religious heads and secular leaders foresee from several angles. The major criteria those are taken into greater consideration are high and elevated landscape, availability of perennial water source nearby and sufficient virgin forest having luxuriant growth all around. Which must provide adequate land for slash and burn type of shifting cultivation, seasonal forest products, materials for house construction and grazing ground for their cattle.

From the structural design and placement of houses one can witness the evidence of social solidarity and oneness feeling among the Kutia Kondh. Two rows of attached houses, across a rectangular space, face each other. All the Kutia Kondh houses of a village maintain on single roof-ridge along a single row. Although each house has its partitioning wall, *verandah* runs continuously from one end to the other. The houses are of almost same type but may vary in size from one group to the other which depends on the economic condition and number of family members of the household. Number of houses vary from 5 to 50 and built on steep hill sides flatten to a gentle slope. The village street is quite wide, neat and clean and at the middle *Meriah* pole is installed before which *Dharani Penu* (*Wangu Penu*), Earth goddess is enshrined. The street is always situated in east-west direction.

In each village, at least one Domb house is usually located a little apart in back side of the settlement. The cowsheds are situated close to the settlement but at the back of hutments. Other hutments are boys' and girls' dormitory in a village which is just like any other typical Kutia Kondh house.

The house construction among the Kutia Kondh involves traditional technique, village co-operative efforts, division of labour and prescribed ritualistic observances. A house may be constructed in a new site when the old settlement is abandoned or in the same settlement when family members are increased due to addition of members by marriage and unable to be accommodated there.

They prefer to live as a well-knit cohesive group in a village where houses are built in one continuous row in east-west direction and at the middle of the village deity is installed.[28] Kutia Kondh is the weakest section leading an isolated life of purity.

The economic life of the Kutia Kondh is largely influenced by the development in the forest environment. Starting from the birth up to the death, all happenings in-between are directly or indirectly linked with forest. The forest provides them with food, cloth and materials for construction of houses. They exploit the forest resources to supplement income from agriculture and horticulture. They also collect house-building materials and herbal medicines from the forest. When time permits, they also go for hunting though it is not regular practice. All over the year, Kutia Kondhs collect varieties of mushrooms, green leaves, shoots, tubers and roots, stems, flowers, fruits, seeds and kernels from the forest in their respective growing seasons. All these were abundantly available in the past and even today they depend on these collections to a large extent. In the lean period many of them absolutely depend on certain nutritive tubers, the availability of which has gone down due to devastation of forest. However, in the summer months they depend on *mahua* flower, mango and tubers and in the early rainy season they eat mango kernels and bamboo shoots along with several green leaves and mushrooms. The Kutia Kondh boys and girls from their late childhood become acquainted with several forest plants and products which are used by them in different ways. As they spend most of their time in forest they get ample opportunity to develop their knowledge in this line. Collection of *lac* gum, honey, hill broom, fibre, leaf for the preparation of cups and plates are occasional works which pay good cash to the Kutia Kondh.[29]

They are generally shifting cultivators. Their lands are divided into back-yard land, up-land, and low land. They grew crops like millets, cereals, turmeric, ginger, mustard, black-gram, arrowroot etc. They follow very simple method of cooking and they usually prepare food like ragi-gruel, vegetable curry and dry-fish. Everybody, irrespective of sex, consume liquor as a social necessity. Tobacco is very commonly used.[30] Kutias, who live in isolation on hill tracts have only a rudimentary knowledge about the modern concept of health and nutrition. There are two micro-projects for the development of Kutia Kondh such as KKDA (Kutia Kondh Development Agencies) functioning one at Belghar in Tumudibandh block, Kandhamala district, established in 1978 and another in Lanjigarh in Kalahandi district, established in 1986.[31]

Food and dietary habit of the Kutia Kondh are influenced by the environment as a whole. Diet routine of the people varies according to season and economic condition of the household. But in general they take three times a day, i.e., morning, mid-day and in the late evening. Meals comprise of ragi-grul, maize, millet and paddy rice, green leaves and vegetables as well as dry fish and meat. Apart from those multifarious edibles, mushrooms, roots, shoots, leaves, flowers, fruits and seeds are also eaten as per availability in different seasons. For quite a long time from late summer up to end of the rains, Kutia Kondhs depend on yam, tubers, bamboo shoots, jack-fruits, *mahua* flower, mango and its kernel.

They do not drink milk and eat eggs. Pork is not eaten by females. The emerging youths of both sexes have given up eating beef. During pregnancy a few food taboos are observed. Children are not given any special diet. No doubt that people in the area specially the poor Kutia Kondhs suffer from diseases related to vitamin deficiency and are in need of nutritive food items. During lean period rice is made available by the government and the Micro Project is encouraging them to raise various vegetable crops.

The Kutia Kondhs take their own brewed rice beer, *mahua* liquor and *sago*-palm sap. They usually consume rice beer brewed out of small millets and the same is used for magico-religious purpose. They also use various narcotics like tobacco leaf powder and paste. Some herbal medicines are mixed in rice beer and *sago*-palm-juice to make these intoxicants.

The Kutia Kondhs as an endogamous unit have their distinct language, territory and style of life. Social organisation among the Kutia Kondhs involves the whole network of social and religious spheres between different individuals and groups. There are groupings among them for several social purposes. It is reflected in behavioural pattern of the individuals and groups within the social framework. Each group may be identified by kinship ties and modes of conduct in general.[32] Kutia Kondh women have their distinct status. They are tabooed from certain religious, traditional and administrative functions but their economic status is very high. They are not permitted to participate in the village council. There are mainly two things which a Kutia Kondh woman must not do, viz. (i) she should not plough the land and (ii) she should not climb the roof of the house for thatching. Hair dressing and bodily deformation with some tattoo marks are some native practices. Certain materials used by the Kutia Kondhs are symbols of self identity e.g., palm-leaf knitted head-band, special lead necklaces etc. Forest products collected by the women are sold in the markets or cooperative societies for cash.[33]

They enjoy the life to the possible extent. They are very free and frank to the known persons and spontaneous in action.

One can easily recognise their fellow feeling and bravery. They are good hosts and try to satisfy the guests in all possible ways. A Kutia Kondh never gets angry with someone and begs before anybody if he is at fault. He believes in work and worship. The Kutia Kondhs trust the Dombs, people of Scheduled Caste community. They never disregard or misbehave anybody unless they are very seriously hurt. They believe in love and affection, excuse and forgiving, help and tolerance. They dislike cheating, characterless and ill-tempered persons. They are afraid of evil spirits, black magicians, sorcerers and touts having long hands with the Government officials. The Kutia Kondhs are disciplined people and bear high sense of morality. They respect elders and love younger ones. For them, physical punishment and use of taunting remarks to somebody are the worst means for sorting out any problem. They never like persons having stealing and begging habit. They are very innovative and imaginative. They believe more in equality than in individual status symbol. They are very sympathetic and helpful at the time of danger. They may tolerate anything but not against their land, people, spirits and culture.[34]

Dongria Kondh

Dongria Kondh is separate from all other sections for their skill in horticulture. They mostly inhabit in the Niyamgiri hill ranges situated in Bissamcuttack and Muniguda Blocks of Gunpur subdivision and Kalyansingpur Block of Rayagada subdivision in Rayagada district and Biswanathpur area of Lanjigarh Block in Kalahandi district. Their habitat is confined to a rectangular forest area situated at a height ranging from 1000 ft. to 5000 ft. above the sea level. As the Dongria Kondh villages are found on the top of hills, they are called by the local plainsmen as the Dongria (the hill dwelling) Kondh. They speak a language known as *Kuvi* with an admixture of Telugu. Their unique characteristic features and rich cultural heritage distinguish them from the neighbouring tribes and non-tribal groups. Their distinctiveness is revealed specially from their dress style, mode of living, indigenous skills and technology, cultural pattern and social system. They claim themselves to be the descendants of the Niyam Raja, their legendary ancestral king. This belief binds them together and keeps their social affinity undisturbed. They are an endogamous group and follow clan exogamy. In recent years, some of them have established matrimonial relations with the neighbouring Desia Kondh community whom they consider as their brothers.

One of the striking characteristic features of the Dongria Kondh is their strong belief in the supernatural power. They attach more importance to group solidarity and ensure it by their sincere devotion to numerous gods, goddesses and spirits. They like hard work and derive pleasure by performing dance and music in their leisure time. They believe in magic, witchcraft and sorcery. In their society, the division of labour on the basis of age and sex is clearly defined and unity among clans is quite strong. The elders are respected and obeyed by the juniors.[35]

These people are extremely laborious and are tenacious about their rights over their land. They are skilled in banana plantation and turmeric cultivation. But one of the drawbacks is their dependence on the local Domb merchants for the purpose of the marketing of their products. There is a symbolic relationship between the Dongrias and the Dombs which cuts across economic activities. Both the communities have been living together since earliest times. Even though the Dongrias feel the cruelty of exploitation they have no other ways but to endure it with limitless patience in the present circumstances because of their illiteracy and ignorance.[36]

The Dongria Kondh villages are situated amidst hills and forests of the Niyamgiri hill ranges. Throughout the year, the area looks green and picturesque. Due to lack of proper communication, many of the villages remain away from the mainstream of the civilisation. All over the hills here and there, one can look at cleared patches without any vegetation ready for slash and burn type shifting cultivation which is not only an age-old practice but also mainstay of their subsistence economy. Apart from these, there are plenty of pineapple, banana, lemon, orange and other plantations as well as jackfruits and mango groves found throughout the area. Adjacent to the villages, sago-palm trees not only add to the scenery but also provide the most favourite traditional drinks to the Dongria Kondh.

The dress and ornaments which adorn Dongria particularly their members distinguish them from other sections of the tribe. In general a Dongria male puts a narrow scarf wrapped around the waist and adorns his body with ornaments of various types. He shaves his head keeping a tuft of hair nearly tied to a knot at the back. Sometimes a leaf rolled cigar is seen tucked in the hair knot at the back. Invariably every Dongria male carries an axe in his waist belt.[37]

Dongria women have no right over her husband's property, only she can work and enjoy. Women are considered to be assets of the family. They help their male folk in weeding, sowing and harvesting. Men and women help each other at the time of need and hardship.[38]

Each Dongria Kondh village has the institution of youth dormitory. It is the centre where unmarried girls spend their leisure time. The number of dormitories varies from village to village. Boys from other villages belonging to different clans visit the girls dormitory and spend nights with the girls. The boys and girls also get chance to interact with one another for choosing their life partners. The dormitory is the cultural centre for various activities of the boys and girls. By and large, it is a place for dance, merrymaking, enjoyment and learning things that become useful in future.

Like the girl's dormitory in every village, there is a community house popularly known as the *Sadar*. The house is constructed on communal labour and cooperation and here community level matters are discussed. Entrance to this house is strictly prohibited for women.

The Dongria Kondhs have an intimate relationship with their forest. It provides them materials for construction of their houses. It serves as the major source of food and other essential consumable items. They collect a variety of mushrooms, tubers, roots, stems, green leaves, flowers, fruits and seeds from the forest. It is the place where their gods, goddess, and spirits live. One cannot think of a complete life of Dongria Kondh without forest.

Apart from forest, they also depend on land for their survival. Their cultivable lands can broadly be classified into three categories, viz. *dongar*, *bhata* and *bada*. *Dongar* means the hill slope land for shifting cultivation where they grow pineapple, citrus plants, banana, turmeric, ginger and varieties of other crops. *Bhata* is a type of land which is situated at the base of the hills which is comparatively more fertile than the *dongar* land. In *bhata* land they mostly take up wet cultivation. The third category of land is the kitchen garden, locally known as *bada* which is kept more fertile by manuring. It is mostly used for growing different types of vegetables. The type of soil of this area is red stony, clay and in some places patches of black soil and red soil are also noticed.

Dongria houses are thatched with grass and the walls are made of wattle and plastered with mud. The roof is so low that the walls are practically invisible from outside and one has to stoop down to get into the house.[39] They also raise livestock. The food pattern is similar to that of the Kutia Kondh. A barter system is still the traditional method for exchanging goods. The women beautify themselves with hairpins, earrings, nose rings and necklaces. But they do not have tattoos. Both females and males grow their hair long which is tied in a knot at the nape of their neck in a traditional fashion.

In the Dongria Kondh society, the family is the smallest basic social unit. There are nuclear as well as joint families which are either monogamous or polygamous. In joint and extended families, several brothers live together with their spouses and children under the care of grandparents. Many Dongria Kondh males prefer to have more than one wife because of economic necessity. Beyond family and lineage there are larger agnatic descent groups, called *Punja*, the maximal lineage. The names of the *Punjas* are *Mandal Punja, Bismajhi Punja, Jani Punja* and *Pujari Punja*.

The clan plays quite vital role in possession and utilisation of land and forest which are two very important productive assets of the Dongria Kondh. Each clan (*Kuda*) has its own territory well demarcated from all sides. The clans belonging to *mutha* have absolute rights over their respective territories. Each *mutha* is composed of clans and each clan of several villages, the number of which vary from one *mutha* to the other.[40]

Dongria Kondhs are neither health conscious nor careful of their health. Even when they are sick, they either work or stroll. But only in acute stage, they seek for treatment. The acute stage is only ascribed due to wrath of the deities and spirits. Normally when indigenous efforts are failed, they prefer allopathic medicines.[41] Development is going on among these people through the Dongria Kondh Development Agency (DKDA) established by the Government one at Kurli, Chatikona block, Gunpur sub-division, Rayagada district, established in the year 1978 and the other at Parasali, Kalyansinghpur block, Rayagada district, established in the year 1987.

Desia Kondh

Desia Kondhs are one of the advanced tribal sections of Kondhs. Their population comprises about 39.4 per cent of the total Kondh population. The Desia Kondhs have left their hills and settled down in plains to pursue cultivation. They inhabit mainly the plains and coastal areas with other non-tribes and follow the Hindu way of living. They are plain agriculturists and have better scope to develop their land by using fertilisers and insecticides. With the irrigation prospects, they produce short duration paddy as well as other agricultural products. Desia Kondhs are more advanced as compared to other sections of Kondhs because of the influence and reach of various developmental activities carried out by the Government.

The Desia Kondhs have completely forgotten *Kui* or *Kuvi*, which is the mother tongue of the Kondh and they speak *Odia* like their *Odia* neighbours. The Desia Kondhs have changed culturally. For example, in the olden days a human being was sacrificed on the occasion of *meriah*. After the human sacrifice was stamped out, the human being was replaced by a buffalo and with it the name of the festival changed from *meriah* to *kedu*. At present most of the Desia kondhs manage the festival with a goat or cock instead of buffalo. In such places the term *kedu* has been replaced by another form i.e., *jantal*.[42]

The Desia Kondh house is very simple. The walls are made of planks of the *Sal* trees covered with mud and the trellis made of bamboo splits are hatched with grass. The layout of the house consists of a bedroom (*dapanidu*), a kitchen (*bajanidu*) and a shed (*gaheli*). A narrow *verandah* is provided in the front as well as in the back of the house.

Desia Kondh women like to wear coloured saris and blouses. Red and blue are their favourite colours. They use different types of ornaments made of beads available in the local markets. Tattooing is most common among these women. They get their faces, hands and legs tattooed with line and dotted with geometrical designs.[43] Dormitories (*dhangadabas*) play an important role in the marital life of the Desia Kondh. Before marriage the young boys choose their life partners from *dinda ghar* or *dhangidi idu*. *Dinda ghar* is meant for young unmarried girls. The young unmarried girls used to spend night in this house.[44]

There has been a gradual change in the institutions of traditional tribal council and dormitory system. These have completely disappeared in the Desia village. This however attacked their traditional value system. They gradually in a sense modernised their own traditional institutions which were given once upon a time great significance.

Desia Kondhs practice four types of cultivation, viz. (i) shifting cultivation on the hill-slopes and hill tops, (ii) *dahi* cultivation on the flat hill tops and at the foot of hills, (iii) dry and low land cultivation and (iv) backyard cultivation. The economic life of the Desia's and their struggle for earning a livelihood mainly centre on agriculture. Collection of edible roots, tubers and leaves from forests, hunting of wild animals, fishing in the hill streams and tanks and water logged paddy fields and wage earnings by daily labour supplement their income from land. The important forest collections include timber, firewood, bamboo, *siali* creepers, *kendu* leaf, *sal* leaf etc.[45]

According to the census of 2001, the total scheduled tribe population in Odisha is 81, 45,081, among them 40, 66,783 is male and 40, 78,298 is female. And the population of Kondh is 13, 95,643 out of which 68, 84, 02 are males and rest are females. Though their population is unevenly spread throughout the state, their main concentration is in south Odisha which comprises the present districts of Ganjam, Gajapati, Kandhamala, Boudh, Koraput, Rayagada, Nabarangapur and Malkangiri.

The district of Ganjam derives its name from the word *Ganj-i-am* which means the granary of the world. The district is named after the old township and European fort. Ganjam situated on the northern bank and near the mouth of the river Rushikulya. Spreading over an area of 8206 sq. km., it is surrounded by Kandhamala in the north-west, Nayagarh in the north, Khurda in the north-east, Gajapati district in the west and the Bay of Bengal in south-east. On its southern periphery the district borders the state of Andhra Pradesh. Ganjam district extends from 19°4′ north latitude to 20°17′ north latitude and 84°7′ east longitude to 85°12′ east longitude.

The physiography of Ganjam gives a perfect platform for the tribals in sustaining their ethno-cultural identity in the district. Forest area covers an area of 315000 ha., out of which 92228.98 ha. consists of reserve forest. The tribal community comprises 2.88 per cent of the total population in Ganjam. The district is home land of various tribal communities. The Kondhs and its subsection constitute the major percentage (49.33) of tribal population in the district.[46]

The district of Gajapati was formed in 1993. It lies between 18°45′ to 19°40′ north latitude and in between 83°5′ to 84°25′ east longitude. The district is bounded by Ganjam on the east and a part in the north. On the north-west border is the Kondhamala and on the west lays the Rayagada district. The entire south of the district is surrounded by the Srikakulam district of Andhra Pradesh which also encircles a bit of the eastern boundary of the district. The major part of the district is hilly and undulated topography. A major proportion of its population is backward particularly schedule tribes. The schedule tribes account for 50.78 per cent population of the district and Shabar (50.84 per cent), Saura (32.21 per cent) and Kondh (14.86 per cent) are the largest tribal groups in the district.[47]

The name of the district Kandhamala is derived from the name of its major inhabitants Kondhs. They were in these hilly tracts before the advent of Aryans. They have been classified under the ancient Gondid race of the Proto-Australoid group, which according to scholars like Risley, preceded the Aryans by many thousand years.

The present Kandhamala district has been carved out of the erstwhile Boudh-Phulabani district, consisting of one subdivision Kandhamala. It is one of the centrally located districts of Odisha and lies between 19°45′ and 20°30′ north latitude and 83°45′ and 84°30′ east longitude. The district is bounded by Boudh in the north, Rayagada, Gajapati and Ganjam on the south, Nayagarh and Ganjam in the east and Kalahandi and Bolangir on the west. The district has an area of 8021 sq. km. with a population of 6.48 lakhs. The schedule tribe population is 51.96 per cent of total population and among the schedule tribes Kondhs only constitute 93.33 per cent of total tribal population in the district.[48]

Boudh was a subdivision of previous undivided district of Phulabani. This enjoyed the status of a district vide Notification No. DRC 218/93-56413 dated 22.12.1993. The district is named after its headquarters town, Boudh, a place located near the bank of river Mahanadi. It is one of the centrally located districts of Odisha and lies between 20° 22′ north and 20°50′ north latitude and between 83° 34′ east and 84°49′ east longitude. It is bounded on the north by the district of Sonepur and Anugul, on the east by Anugul and Nayagarh, on the south by Nayagarh and Kandhamala and on the west by Bolangir and Sonepur. The area of the district is 3098 sq. km. with a population of 373372 (2001 Census). The district population is constituted by 21.88 per cent of schedule castes and 12.47 per cent of schedule tribes. The major tribes enumerated in the district are Kondh, Gond, Soura etc. and Kondhs only comprise 76.44 per cent of total tribal population of the district.[49]

Koraput district is full of natural beauty, which fills one's heart with immense joy. This district has a rich geographical diversity abounding stupendous hills, dense forest, wild meadows, picturesque waterfalls, terraced valleys and eternal springs. It retains the title conferred on her by her admirers as the "Paradise of Odisha" or as "Darjeeling of Odisha". The district headquarters is situated at an altitude of 96 mt. above the sea level. This level of nature's abundance has been the home to Odisha's vast primitive and ethnic tribal population.

The district is located between 18° and 19° north latitude and 82° and 83° east longitude in the extreme southern part of Odisha. It is bounded by Rayagada and Srikakulum (A. P.) in the east, Malkangiri and Bastar (M.P.) in the west, Nabarangapur and Rayagada in the north and Vizianagaram and Vizag (A.P.) in the south. The district has an area of 8807 sq. km. with a population of 11.8 lakhs (2001 Census). The schedule tribes account for 49.62 per cent population of the district and Kondh (28.71 per cent), Paraja (30.08 per cent) and Bhottada (10.78 per cent) are the major tribal groups in the district.[50]

Rayagada is one of the beautiful districts of Odisha. The natural beauty of this place always captivates one's mind. The charming valleys of the river Nagavali and Vansadhara, vast stretches of hills, ever green forests, perennial streams, stiff and massive rocks standing like mythological demons and deep holes in the rocky river beds presenting thrilling sights are the attractive features of the district. According to local people, the name Rayagada has been derived from *Raya* means rock, *Gadda* means deep holes, which signifies deep holes in the rocks.

The district is located between 19° and 19°58′ north latitude and 82°5′ and 84°2′ east longitude in southern part of Odisha. It is bounded by Gajapati district in the east, Koraput and Kalahandi in the west, Kondhamala in the north and Koraput and Srikakulum (A.P.) in south. As per 2001 Census the district having 7073 sq. km. of geographical area has 8 lakh of population. The schedule tribes account for 55.76 per cent population of the district and Kondh alone constitute 71.09 per cent of total tribal population.[51]

The district of Nabarangapur, with her golden autumn and mystery morning of the monsoon months, her painted spring and slumbering summer and her winter ranging from fierce to mild, provides varieties of livings in different seasons, which is rare elsewhere. The district derives its name from its headquarters town Nabarangapur.

It is located between 19°9′ and 20°5′ north latitude and 81°52′ and 82°53′ east longitude. The district is bounded by Chhattisgarh in the west and north, by Kalahandi district in the east and Koraput in the south. It has a geographical area of 5291 sq. km. The population of the district as per 2001 Census is 10 lakhs. The schedule tribes comprising various tribal communities constitute 55.03 per cent of total population in the district and among the schedule tribes Kondhs constitute 8.96 per cent of total tribal population of the district.

Malkangiri district is full of natural beauty. Long range hills, dense forests, rivers, streams, reservoir and waterfalls are the major attractions of this district. On the whole, the landscape of the district presents a scenic beauty. It is believed by the local people that the name Malkangiri has been derived from the name of a hill "Malyabanta giri". It is situated between 81°24' and 82°25′ east longitude and 17°49′ and 18°44′ north latitude in the extreme southern part of Odisha. It is bounded by Koraput district on the north, East Godavari of Andhra Pradesh on the south, Visakhapatnam district of Andhra Pradesh on the east and Bastar district of Chhattisgarh on the west. The district covers a geographical area of 5791 sq. km. As per 2001 Census the total population of the district is 5.04 lakhs. The long range hills and dense forests are homeland to some primitive tribal communities and as per 2001 Census data the tribes constitute 57.43 per cent of total population in the district.[52] Among the schedule tribe population Kondhs comprise 6.22 per cent of the total tribal population.

Thus Kondh population is mostly concentrated in the southern part of Odisha. Most of the part of Kondh territory is excessively hilly, and the central table land has an elevation of about 2000 feet above the sea level. While some portions of the territory are quite bereft of wood, others are covered with thickly clustered trees. At the foot of the hills are found bamboo forest. The climate of the Kondh territories is highly insalubrious.[53] The rivers of the Kondh tracts pose a liability for the inhabitants. The river is not useful for irrigation. When the water is needed the river is all about dry and deep down below the steep bank. During the dry season, it is possible to walk over the river bed without getting one's feet wet.[54]

Kondhs are considered as the original inhabitants of India who have carried forward a legacy of rich and distinct cultural traits for many centuries. Their living culture and life style is very much fascinating. Indeed this tribe has many precious cultural traits and incredible heritage. Though the life style of Kondhs has a lot of changes with the march of time, yet they have not given up their customs traditions, beliefs and outstanding traditional knowledge. There is a need to know about them and preserve their socio-cultural identities.

Table-1 shows the Kondh inhabited area in the state.

Table 1: Kondh Inhabited Areas in Odisha

Sl. No	*Zones/Regions*	*Area Covered*
1.	Northern Zone	Sundargarh, Keonjhar and Mayurbhanj districts. Bamra and Kuchinda portion of Sambalpur district, Interior plains of Balasore district and pallahara region of Dhenkanal district.
2.	Central Zone	Whole of the Brahmani and the Baitarani basins.
3.	Eastern Ghat Region	
4.	(i) Northern section	Starting from Nilgiri in Balasore district stretches up to border in Puri district.
	(ii) Central section	Boudh, Balliguda, G. Udaygiri areas of Phulbani district.
	(iii) Rayagada section	Paralakhemundi areas of Gajapati district and Rayagada district.
	(iv) South eastern section	Areas of Pattangi section of Koraput district.
	(v) Malkangiri section	Area of Malkangiri district.
	(vi) South western section	Plains area and Dongara area of Kalahandi district.
	(vii) Coastal region	Eastern seaboard plains stretching from the mouth of the Rushikulya river to the Subarnarekha river.

Source: The Kandha of Orissa, SCSTRTI, Bhubaneswar, 2006, 309.

Table 2: Scheduled Caste and Scheduled Tribe Population of South Odisha.

Sl. No.	*District*	*Population*	*Geographical area in sq. km*	*SC*	*ST*
1.	Boudh	317622	3444.8	62377	41022
2.	Kandhamala	456281	5464.9	99499	281386
3.	Ganjam	2704056	8070.6	484187	79120
4.	Gajapati	454708	3016.8	39898	217725
5.	Koraput	1029986	8379.3	138169	521849
6.	Malkangiri	421917	6115.3	84208	246214
7.	Nabarangapur	846659	5290	127800	467919
8.	Rayagada	713984	7584.7	101956	400097

Source: Census of India-2001, Directorate of Census, Bhubaneswar.

Table 2 reveals SC and ST population and inhabited geographical area of different districts of south Odisha.

Table 3: Kondh Population of Different Districts of South Odisha, Male/Female, Rural/Urban wise.

Sl. No.	*Name of District*	*Total Kondh Population Male / Female*	*Total Kondh Population in Rural Area Male / Female*	*Total Kondh Population in Urban Area Male / Female*
1.	Koraput	168172 83403 (M) 84769 (F)	166927 82680 (M) 84247 (F)	1245 723 (M) 522 (F)
2.	Malkangiri	15503 7679 (M) 7824 (F)	15316 7568 (M) 7748 (F)	187 111 (M) 76 (F)
3.	Nabarangapur	42095 20974 (M) 21121 (F)	41911 20859 (M) 21052 (F)	184 115 (M) 69 (F)
4.	Rayagada	329461 159224 (M) 170237 (F)	322668 155961 (M) 166707 (F)	6793 3263 (M) 3530 (F)

contd...

Sl. No.	*Name of District*	*Total Kondh Population Male/Female*	*Total Kondh Population in Rural Area Male/ Female*	*Total Kondh Population in Urban Area Male/ Female*
5.	Ganjam	44850 22407 (M) 22443 (F)	43690 21806 (M) 21884 (F)	1160 601 (M) 559 (F)
6.	Gajapati	39164 18918 (M) 20246 (F)	39103 18883 (M) 20220 (F)	61 35 (M) 26 (F)
7.	Boudh	35587 17789 (M) 17798 (F)	35282 17626 (M) 17656 (F)	305 163 (M) 142 (F)
8.	Kandhamala	314355 155266 (M) 159089 (F)	308845 152467 (M) 156378 (F)	5510 2799 (M) 2711 (F)
9.	South Odisha as a whole	989187 485660 (M) 503527 (F)	973742 477850 (M) 495892 (F)	15445 7810 (M) 7635 (F)
10.	Odisha as a whole	1395643 688402 (M) 707241 (F)	1363137 671651 (M) 691486 (F)	32506 16751 (M) 15755 (F)

Source: *Census of India-2001*, Directorate of Census, Bhubaneswar.

Table 3 reflects the Kondh population of different districts of south Odisha, male/female wise and rural/urban wise. From the table it is evident that the population of the Kondhs in Odisha as per the Census of India 2001 is 13, 95,643 (male- 6, 88,402, female- 7, 07,241). The sex ratio favours the females i.e., 1027 females per thousand males. This is one of the important indicators of the higher status of women in their society.

Table 4: Growth Rate of Kondh Population in Odisha

Year	*Population*	*Growth*	*Growth Rate*
1931	5,93,900	–	–
1941	6,90,305	96,375	16.23
1951	7,54,606	64,241	8.51
1961	8,18,847	64,241	8.51
1971	8,69,965	51,118	6.24
1981	9,89,342	1,19,377	13.72
1991	11,40,374	1,51,032	15.27
2001	13,95,643	2,55,269	22.38

Source: Census of India 1931-2001, Directorate of Census, Bhubaneswar.

Table 4 reveals that the Kondh population is showing faster growth rate since 1981. This community is one of the well-known tribal groups of India in the state of Odisha.

References

1. P.K.V. Kaimal (ed.), *Encyclopedia of India*, Vol. V, *Orissa*, Rima Publishing House, New Delhi, 1992, p. 1.
2. *Ibid.*, p. 4.
3. Almas Ali, "Heath Status of Tribals in India: An Overview", in Dipak Kumar Adak, Biswanath Bhattacharya, Rohini Ghosh, Manoranjan Pal, Premanand Bharati and T.S. Vasulu, (eds.), *Demography and Health Profile of Tribals*, Anmol Publication, New Delhi, 2003, p. 2.
4. P.K. Nayak, "Social, Cultural and Linguistic Variations in Tribal Orissa: Tribes of Orissa", Schedule Castes and Schedule Tribes Research and Training Institute (herein after SCSTRTI), Bhubaneswar, 2004, p. 1.
5. P.K. Mohanty, *Encyclopedia of Schedule Tribes in India*, Vol. 4, East, Isha Books, Delhi, 2006, pp. 142-144.
6. P.K. Dalai, *Life and Culture of the Kondha Tribe in Orissa*, Unpublished Thesis, submitted to Berhampur University, 2003, p. 2.
7. N. Patnaik and P.S. Das Patnaik, *The Kondhs of Orissa*, Tribal and Harijan Research-cum-Training Institute, (herein after THRTI), Bhubaneswar, 1982, pp. i-x.
8. N. Patnaik, *Kondh* (ed.), SCSTRTI, Bhuabaneswar, 1989, pp. 2–3.

9. *Ibid.,* p. 3.
10. Bijay Kumar Behera, *Tribal Culture, Modernisation and Development, A Study of Kondh Tribe*, Khama Publisher, New Delhi, 1996, p. 26.
11. N.R. Patnaik, *History and Culture of Kondh Tribes*, Commonwealth Publishers, New Delhi, 1992, 10-11
12. *Ibid.,* pp. 11-13.
13. N. Patnaik *op cit.*, pp. 3-4.
14. N.R. Patnaik, *op. cit.*, pp. 15-16.
15. A.L. Basham, *The Wonder That was India,* New York, Vol.1, 1959, p. 53.
16. N. Patnaik, *op.cit.*, p. 3.
17. *The Kandha of Orissa*, SCSTRTI, Bhubaneswar, 2006, xii- xiii.
18. N.R. Patnaik, *op. cit.,* 17-18.
19. Krishan Shrama, *The Konds of Orissa*, Concept Publishing Company, New Delhi, 1979, p. p. 17.
20. T.J. Maltby, *Ganjam Manual,* Madras, 1918, 55.
21. R.C.S. Bell, *Orissa District Gazetteer, Koraput*, 1945, p. 66.
22. Verrier Elwin, *A Brief Survey of The Aboriginal Tribes of The District of Ganjam and Koraput,* Cuttack, 1946, p. 34.
23. T.J. Maltby, *Ganjam Manual,* Madras, 1918, p. 55.
24. G.F. Paddison, *Partially Excluded Report,* submitted to Madras Government, 1916, p. 91.
25. Krishana Shrama, *The Kondha of Orissa, op., cit.*, p. xii.
26. G. Bulliya, "Habitat, Health and Nutrition problems of Kondhs", in Vijay S. Sahay and Pradip Kumar Singh (eds.), *Dimensions of Research in Indian Anthropology*, Vol. I, Serial Publications, New Delhi, 2003, p. 333.
27. Sarat Chandra Mohanty, "The Kandha of Kandhamalas During British Raj," *Adivasi*, Vol. 48, No. 1, June, 2008, p. 61.
28. G. Bulliyya, *op., cit.*, pp. 332-333.
29. *Development Hand Book for the Kutia Kondh* of Kutia Kondh Development Agency (K.K.D.A), Belghar, Phulbani District, Government of Orissa, Welfare Department, Government Press, Cuttack, 1996, pp. 22-23.
30. G. Bulliyya, B.V. Babu, S.S.S. Mahapatra, R.N. Nayak, A.S. Kerketta, *Health Status of The Elderly Population Among Four Primitive Tribes of Orissa, India, A Clinico-epidemiological*

Study, A Report of Regional Medical Research Centre (RMRC), Bhubaneswar, 15th July 2007.

31. Kalpana Patnaik, "Kutia Kondh Development Agency (KKDA), Lanjigarh: A Development Profile, *Adivasi*, No. 1, Vol. 48, 2008, SCSTRTI, Bhubaneswar, p. 76.
32. *Development Hand Book for the Kutia Kondh* of Kutia Kondh Development Agency (K.K.D.A), *op. cit.*, p. 28.
33. *Ibid.*, p. 26.
34. *Ibid.*, p. 36.
35. A.C. Sahoo "The Traditions and Customs of the Dongria Kondh of Orissa". in *Adivasi*, Vol. XXXVI, Part-2, June and December, 1996, SCSTRTI, Bhubaneswar, p. 34.
36. N. Patnaik, and P.S. Das Patnaik, *op. cit.,* p. 5.
37. *The Kandha of Orissa*, SCSTRTI, *op. cit.,* p. 3.
38. A.C. Sahoo, *op. cit.*, pp. 36-37.
39. Sitakanta Mahapatra and Nityananda Pattnaik, *Patterns of Tribal Housing*, Academy of Tribal Dialect and Culture, Bhubaneswar, 1986, p. 28.
40. A.C. Sahoo, *op. cit.*, 36.
41. The Kandha of Orissa, SCSTRTI, op. cit., p. 217.
42. *Ibid.*, pp. 309-311.
43. *Ibid.*, p. 316.
44. Chitta Ranjan Mishra, "Dindaghar' and the Marital Tradition of Desia Kondhs in Kondhmala District," in *Orissa Review*, January. 2008, p. 46.
45. P.K. Dalai, *op. cit.*, p. 9.
46. *Orissa Review,* Census Special, December, 2010, p. 112.
47. *Ibid.*, pp. 107-108.
48. *Ibid.*, pp. 131-132.
49. *Ibid.*, pp. 87-88.
50. *Ibid.*, pp. 147-148.
51. *Ibid.*, pp. 175-176.
52. *Ibid.*, pp. 151-152.
53. N.R. Patnaik, *op. cit.,* p. 2.
54. *Ibid.*, p. 7.

2

Concept of Health and Hygiene

Good health is a concern of all living beings. It is a prerequisite for human development and is an essential component for the well being of mankind. Health is wealth. Thus health of an individual is an important aspect for human population and almost becomes a precondition for achieving efficient human resources development. Health is a universally cherished goal. Health cannot be forced upon the people. It is a positive attribute of life and the accessibility of health services to all people is considered to be the key step towards development. Even after half a century of independence of our country much has not been achieved in the area of health in general and for the underprivileged group in particular. Many popular health programmes have been implemented from time to time to meet the special needs of the people at various levels. The tribals have their own distinct and unique cultural milieu and lifestyle. In addition to this they also have many deep rooted practices of indigenous system of health care. Due to a combination of societal attitudes, varying belief system, tribal population throughout Odisha has less access to basic health care.

Health is a state of dynamic equilibrium between the organism and its environment which maintains the structural and functional characteristic of the organism within the normal limit for the particular form of life and particular phase of its life cycle. For all practical purposes the individual can be said to be healthy when he is free from subjective symptoms, objective defects and disease.[1]

Health care is one of the most important of all human endeavours to improve the quality of life especially of the tribal people. Despite remarkable world-wide progress in the field of diagnostics and curative and preventive health, still there are people living in isolation in natural and polluted surroundings far away from civilisation with their traditional values, customs, beliefs and myths intact. They are commonly known as tribals and considered to be autochthonous people of the land.[2] The Kondhs are not different. The health status of the Kondhs is poor and they are facing a lot of health problems because of their isolation, remoteness and lack of health consciousness. Living in isolation on hill tracts, the Kondhs have only a rudimentary knowledge about the modern concept of health and nutrition. Their strong faith on the traditional magico-religious practices is the main reason for their low degree of awareness towards modern medicines and medical practices. Lack of knowledge about environmental sanitation, personal hygiene and poor living condition are some of the major factors responsible for their poor health.[3]

Health is differently interpreted from different perspectives. The bio-medical approach which dominated the medical thought till the end of nineteenth century based on the "germ theory of disease" views health as an 'absence of disease'. The approach almost ignores the role of environmental, psychological and other socio-cultural factors in finding health. The ecological approach views health as a dynamic equilibrium between man and his environment. For them disease is maladjustment of the human organism to environment. The psychological approach states that health is not only related to body but also to mind and especially to the attitude of the individual. The socio-cultural approach considers health as a product of the social and community structure. Health is the priceless asset of a man. It is man's natural condition. It is his birth right. It is the result of living in accordance with natural laws pertaining to body, mind and environment. These laws relate to fresh air, sunlight, diet, exercise, rest, relaxation, sleep, cleanliness, right attitude of mind, good habits and above all lifestyle. To quote the observation of the World Health Organisation,

"Health is a state of complete physical, mental and social well-being and not merely an absence of disease or infirmity." Health is multidimensional. There are three dimensions of health such as physical, mental and social.

Physical Dimension

The state of physical health implies the notion of "perfect functioning of the body". It is conceptualised as a state in which every organ is in perfect harmony with the rest of the body.

Mental Dimension

Good mental health is the ability to respond to the varied experiences of life with flexibility and sense of purpose and proportion. The sign of a mentally healthy person is that he faces problems and solves them intelligently.

Social Dimension

The social dimension of health includes the level of social skills one possesses for social functioning and the ability to see one self as a member of a large society.

The health status of an individual, a community or of a nation is determined by the interplay and integration of two ecological universes, the internal environment of the man himself and the external environment which surrounds him.[4] For forest people, ill health indicates end on a continuum. A tribal considers a healthy person as an individual capable of consuming a variety of seasonal and festive food in good quantities delivering the right amount of work output and participating in socio-cultural functions as well as attending to the usual house-hold chores easily. They do not consider pregnant women, mentally or physically challenged persons and the aged ones as patients.[5]

While there is a broad understanding of the health and nutrition problem of the general population and the rural communities of India, such information on tribal population particularly on Kondhs for that matter is meagre. Studies pertaining to health and nutrition among different tribal groups of India are very few, very patchy and scanty. The mortality rate among the Kondh people is also comparatively higher than the non-tribal population. Wide-spread poverty, illiteracy, malnutrition, inhospitable environment, the absence of sanitary living conditions, ignorance of the causes of maladies and their remedy, lack of health services or inability to seek and use them are considered as the attributing factors for their bad health. To be more specific, the overall health status of the Kondh community is conditioned to the factors like (i) effects of environment where they inhabit, (ii) behavioural pattern and life style, (iii) health care delivering service in the Kondh inhabitant areas and (iv) hereditary and genetic determinants. All these subsystems calculate the totality of the health status of the Kondhs. Therefore the health problem of the Kondhs is as varied as tribal group's themselves.[6]

The health scenario of the Kondhs presents a kaleidoscopic mosaic of various communicable and non-communicable diseases. They still depend primarily on hunting and food gathering as primary source of livelihood. They are still far away from the modern civilisation and developments. In spite of a lot of development in health care they still follow their traditional method of treatment and depend upon magico-religious methods.

The Kondhs who live below poverty line in the interior areas do not pay the required attention to health. General health status of the Kondh is poor as compared to the modern society. They suffer from some distinct health problems not because they have some specific type of health but because of specific placement in different areas and circumstances in which they live.[7]

Studies undertaken in the country indicate that the primitive tribes have distinct health problems mainly governed by multidimensional factors like their habitat, difficult terrain and ecological variable niches like illiteracy, poverty, isolation, superstition and deforestation. Hence an integrated multidisciplinary approach has been adopted by different researchers to study the tribal health problems in case of the Kondhs. Their health problems are not equal; it varies from place to place, because the health status completely depends upon different factors like food habit, water, sanitation, hygiene and environmental condition.

Food Habits

Food, shelter and clothing are the basic needs of every human being. Almost all the tribal people live in forest and mountainous regions. They collect their maximum food stuff from the forest. They get edible tubers, fruits, flowers, leafs, mushrooms, honey or other medicinal plants from it. That is why forest is everything to them.[8] The Kondhs also depend upon forest for medicine. They have irregular food habits. So it is difficult to ascertain their nutritional status. They do not have fixed time for eating. They eat whenever they feel hungry and when food is available. Sometimes they just fill their stomach by eatable forest products like wild fruit, edible roots and wild animal flesh which they obtain by hunting. Their staple food varies from season to season.

The different cereals taken by Kondhs are *ragi*, rice, maize, sanwan and millet. *Ragi* is the staple diet taken throughout the year and in winter season rice is used along with *ragi*. In summer Kondhs use mango kernels as their staple diet. They prepare gruel from mango kernels which have no protein value. The intake of milk and milk product is nil. Even tea is unknown in the interior villages.[9] Kondh eats three times a day i.e. in the morning, in midday and in the night. The morning meal consists of only *ragi*-gruel and a pinch of salt. The same food is taken in midday with cooked green leaves. The night meal comprises either *ragi*-gruel cooked with *kosla* rice or unboiled rice and vegetable curry. The Dongria Kondhs are fond of dry fish. They take it after baking directly on fire. It is usually taken with the night meal. Various creepers like *kating*, *baila* and *jhudunga* are boiled, fried and eaten during winter. Pulses like *Kandula* (red gram) is prepared as *dal*, maize is fried and eaten while working in the farm land. Various roots like *rani- kanda* and *nangal kanda* are boiled and eaten as morning tiffin. Comparably better food is eaten in winter months. Green leaves and mushrooms are eaten more during summer and rainy season. Fish is eaten during summer if there is any catch. Scarcity of food is experienced during lean months. Fruits though available in plenty are not consumed but marketed for ready cash. They take chicken, mutton, buffalo meat, pork and beef. The latter two items are the main food items of festive occasion and marriage ceremonies. Regularity in eating is not maintained throughout the year. When there is heavy pressure of work during sowing and harvesting the women specially skip their tiffin and lunch. The men are also irregular in taking food during agricultural season.[10] Diet pattern is never systematic and standardised. It is observed that pregnant and lactating women are not given extra nutritional food. Rather during pregnancy the mother is not allowed to take meat or any sort of animal flesh. They assume that it may harm the growing fetus.[11]

Their dietary system is shaped by the conditions of forest life and agriculture products. Seasoned cycle in the supply of food articles appears to be the main cause for the approximate, uniformity in the standard of consumption of the Kondhs. Besides this absences of glaring economic disparities in form of family income in the interior Kondh villages explain the situation to a great extent. An interesting thing is that in feast a Kondh can eat rice as much as one *tambi* (one and half kilogram) or more, but in his house this amount is shared by four to five persons. An ordinary meal of an ordinary Kondh consists of one leaf cup of cooked rice or *katinga* or maize or *ragi*, some salt and chilly. Wasting of food is not found among Kondhs. They can go without food for some days at a time. They do not hesitate to take gladly whatever is available to them. Their wants are limited. Poor Kondhs cannot afford three meals a day. So they generally drop the morning meal.[12]

Table 1: Annual Cycle of Food Consumption of the Kondhs

Summer (March, April, May and June)	*Rainy (July, August, September and October)*	*Winter (November, December, January and February)*
Food Consumption		
Mango stone powder, jackfruit seeds are mainly consumed. *Ragi* gruel is occasionally taken. Ripe mangoes, jackfruits, cashew nut and pulses become the major food items. Green leafy vegetables constitute a minor portion of curry.	Acute deficit of food getting, Mango stones powder is prepared as gruel and added with *ragi* if possible, maize, jackfruit seeds are boiled and eaten. Rice, millet, tubers, green leaves, and other vegetables are cooked and consumed.	*Ragi* is mainly eaten. Rice, maize, greens and honey consumed, Various roots, tubers, mushrooms, leaves, meat and wild fruits are collected from the forests and consumed. In each village, social and festive occasions are celebrated in groups with feasts.

Source: G. Bulliyya, "Habitat, Health and Nutritional Problems of Kondhs", in Vijoy S. Sahay and Pradip K. Singh, (eds.), *Dimensions of Researches in Indian Anthropology*, Vol.-I, Serial Publications, New Delhi, 2003, 344.

The above table depicts the cycle of food consumption throughout the year by the Kondhs. This table also explains the limitation concerning their food habits. They are not in a position to consume cereals and pulses throughout the year due to their poor economic condition as well as inaccessible habitation. The intake of various essential constituents of food is nutritionally inadequate and ill balanced.

As forest is decreasing day by day they are not getting their required food materials. The scarcity of food grains sometimes compel them to take different types of food stuff such as the powder of the rotten mango kernels. It proves hazardeous to their health and due to this malnutrition they suffer from anaemia and other diseases.[13] The Kondhs do not eat snakes, lizards and other vermins, the flesh of any carnivorous wild animals, or the flesh of bears and monkeys. All kinds of birds like parrots, doves, peacocks, fowls are eaten.[14]

The Kondhs collect their food materials from the forests as mentioned below.

(i) Fruits: *Amba, Kendu, Panasa, Annala, Koliari, Amli-fala, Ankle-kuli, Koting-koli* and *Podi-koli.*

(ii) Green leaves: *Girli, Koliari-kuchha, Jaba-kuchha, Kopu-kuchha, Koti-kuchha, Gandri-kuchha, Barada-kuchha, Mali-kuchha, Kanta-hopka-kuchha, Chhatu-kuchha, Chhakunda-kuchha, Mederenga-kuchha, Kena-kuchha* and *Khiprti-kuchha.*

(iii) Roots and tubers: *Rani-kanda, Nangal-kanda, Pita-kanda, Seabil-kanda, Saru-kanda, Chaul-saru-kanda, Thoda-kanda, Khajrana-saru-kanda, Alu-kanda* and *Rang saru-kanda.*

(iv) Mushrooms: *Amba-chati, Pansa-chati, Sargi-chati, Basa-chati, Kupu-chati, Manei-chati, Surubali-chati, Phuli-chati, Piyal-chati, Dung-chati, Medrenga-chati, Dakel-chati, Ghusra-chati, Mayurbandh-chati, Jambu-chati, Tak-chati, Kun-chati* and *Banj-chati.*

(v) Honey: *Bichhana, Satpuria, Dummi* and *Bagh* are the names of different bees and honey is named after different hives.

(vi) Birds: *Pandka* (Pigeon), *Kugure* (Dove), *Sari* (Myna), *Kirang* (Parrot), *Kaju* (Jungle fowl) and *Milu* (Peacock) are caught and prepared as special dish.

(vii) Animals: *Sibda (Sambara), Kotra (Kutra), Mralu* (Rabbit) and *Sranki* (Porcupine) are hunted for special dishes.[15]

While fruits are plenty in summer, green leaves and mushrooms are available during rainy season. The lean period starts from May and ends in August, when the little millet and maize are mature. Lean period is precarious for the Kondhs as they live on rice stocked earlier and on finger millet from which they prepare gruel. To supplement their diet the *Kutia's* search for mango kernels, *sago* wild and cultivated tubers (*basanga*). It is not uncommon for the *Kutia* families to suffer from hunger during lean period. Diseases are rife as a result of malnutrition. In the rainy season, the Kondhs depend on bamboo shoots called *terka* in Kui language. Those are cut into fine chips. These chips are first ground then squeezed to remove water and they cook it with rice. Fine chips of bamboo are also cooked with pulses or vegetables. Towards the end of rainy season maize matures in shifting cultivation and this saves the people from hunger or even starvation. The most affluent period for the Kondhs is the harvest and the lean period is rainy season. Many other varieties of wild banana flowers, piths of sago palm, pith of the banana plant are also eaten by the Kondhs.[16]

Food is the basic necessity for survival and life cannot exist without food. Food has a quantitative aspect relating to food supply and consumption and a qualitative aspect provided by nutrients which it contains. Nutrition can very well be considered as one of the most important environmental factors affecting the health of all human beings. The Kondhs are no exception to it. Nutrition and diet are not synonyms though they are popularly used in that fashion. Diet consists of various articles of food which are ingested and converted for use in the body for building up and maintaining it in a vital condition. Nutrition is the end of the process by which these are assimilated and the desired result is produced. Man's physical development and growth, his capacity and fitness to work can be considerably improved by means of better nutrition. Malnutrition means a person who does not get food which has all the nutrients, what his body requires. All those who are under-nourished are naturally malnourished.[17]

It is revealed from various studies that the diet of some of the tribals of Odisha is inadequate to the accepted standard, both in quality and quantity. Basic calorie requirements are not met,and intake of protein is very marginal while intake of vitamins and minerals falls far short to the desirable level.[18] The survey made in Kondh villages shows that a high incidence of disease is caused by nutritional deficiency. Thus among the health hazards their nutritional deficiency diseases occupy a unique place. The real cause of early death of most of the Kondh children is the underlying malnutrition.[19]

The average Kondh diet consists of cereals and pulses primarily, which mostly accounts for their calorie intake. In order to assess whether a person suffers from malnutrition, we have to find out the calorie requirement and intake. A calorie is a measure of energy supplied by the food taken. Calorific needs vary with age, sex, weight, physique and environment in which we live in. Even if the body is at rest it needs a certain amount of energy for essential functions such as respiration, circulation and maintenance of body temperature etc. As the Kondhs practise shifting cultivation and the production of food from this source is scarce, there is not sufficient food for the whole year. The cereals and millets hardly last for four months and for the rest eight months they depend on wild roots, tubers, fruits and leaves of edible plants. Consumption of sugar and jiggery is also very rare. The amount and the diet of food intake by the Kondhs is much less than recommended amount and the diet of Kondh is nutritionally more deficient than that of the others. Their food lacks several essential nutrients. Health condition under such gross dietary deficiency can never be satisfactory. As per the Indian Council of Medical Research (I.C.M.R.) report the average calorie intake of an adult Kondh is 1708.9 and this has been calculated from the staple diet of the Kondhs. The caloric value is less than the average Indian quantity i.e. 2100 calories as per the survey report of Krishan Sharma. The total calorie requirement for an adult recommended by I.C.M.R is 2500.[20]

Table 2: Composition of the Average Diet of Kondhs compared with the Average Indian Diet and Indian Council of Medical Research Recommended Diet.

I *Constituent*	*II* *Average Indian Quantity*	*III* *ICMR recommend-ed Quantity*	*IV* *Average Intake of an Adult Kondh*
Protein	58 g.	70 g.	43.24 g.
Fat	29 g.	50 g.	8.57 g.
Carbohydrate	405 g.	440 g.	365.33 g.
Calories	2100	2500	1708.9
Minerals	-	-	13.48 g.
Calcium	0.6 g.	0.8 g.	1.2 g.
Phosphorus	1.3 g.	1.4 g.	1.42 g.
Iron	31 g.	40 mg.	62.7 mg.
Vitamin A	1200 lU	7300 lU	-
Vitamin B1	1.7 mg.	1.8 mg.	-
Vitamin C	5.7 mg.	200 mg.	-
Cereals	471 g.	400 g.	475 g.
Milk	80 g.	170 g.	-
Pulses	68 g.	85 g.	30 g.
Leafy Vegetable	20 g.	116 g.	-
Other vegetable	91 g.	85 g.	-
Oils and fats	14 g.	28 g.	-
Sugar and Jiggery	20 g.	57 g.	-
Meat, fish and eggs	14 g.	28 g.	-
Fruits and nuts	6 g.	57 g.	-
Fruit products	-	-	30 g.

Source: Krishan Sharma, *The Konds of Orissa*, Concept Publishing Company, New Delhi, 1979, 41.

These figures indicate concisely that the Kondhs are under or malnourished with respect to the calorific value of the food articles. The diet survey shows that the kondh diet is inadequate according to accepted standard.

Not only is their food simple but also method of cooking. Salt and turmeric paste are the only condiments used for preparing curry. Garlic, green chilly is added for taste. Garlic, onion, ginger and dry chilly are used when fish or meat curry is prepared. The medium of cooking both vegetarian and non-vegetarian dishes is castor oil. Ground nut oil is used in feast. Fish is cooked mainly with mustard-seeds and chilly. Dry fish is simply baked on fire and eaten along with salt. To make it tasty oil is added sometimes not always. Animals when killed or sacrificed are cooked without being skinned. Mushrooms are soaked in turmeric water before cooking. Anything collected from forest is not directly cooked. The collected stuff is boiled first and then cooked with fresh water.[21] Method of food preparation and cooking is an important factor in determining the level of nutrition we get. It not only adds taste to the food but also adds nutrition which the body needs more. Tribal people of Odisha prefer boiled, baked and roasted food.[22] Kondhs are not much careful about the preparation of food. They even eat some food items raw. They do not always peel off the vegetable and cook it directly after cutting them into small pieces. Before cooking, food materials are not meticulously cleaned and washed. They believe that through washing taste of food items will be reduced. They do not have any concept of vitamin.

As per the survey conducted by the Indian Council Medical Research, it is shown here that how the Kondhs are neglecting their diet. The survey is made among the Dongria Kondhs of Rayagada.

Table 3: Average Consumption of Foodstuffs (g./cu./day) among the Dongria Kondhs of Odisha.

Food stuffs (g)	*Recommended Dietary Intake*	*Dongria Kondh intake*
Cereals and Millets	460 g.	473 g.
Pulses	40 g.	21 g.
Green leafy vegetables	40 g.	11 g.
Roots and tubers	50 g.	52 g.
Other vegetables	60 g.	42 g.
Milk and milk products	150 g.	0
Fats and oils	20 g.	4.8 g.

Sources: A. B. Ota and S. K. Kar, *Ecology of Health and Nutrition Study of Primitive Tribes in Perspective.* A Report of SCSTRTI, Bhubaneswar, under the collaboration of Regional Medical Research Centre, Bhubaneswar, 2006, 20.

The above table shows that the milk and milk products taken by the Kondhs is nil and all other products or food stuff are very marginal than the recommended diet. Only the roots and tubers are more than the recommended value.

Drinking Habits

Although the Kondhs are not too much careful about their diet, they are very much particular about their drinks. They drink either juice collected from *sago*-palm tree or *mohua* liquor in the house of Dombs. The high terrain upon which the *Dongria* Kondhs live, its topography, climate and their living condition force them to be perpetual addicts and make them sometimes wild. Liquor has special charm for them. Except a few, all are habituated to drink and avail any opportunity irrespective of distance of either liquor shop or *sago*-palm trees or condition of the purse. They are so much addicted to it that they can forego their meals. Liquor is locally called *kalu*. Various kinds of liquor brewed by the Dongria Kondhs domestically are:

(i) *Arkhi-kalu* (*Mahua* liquor)

(ii) *Panasa-kalu* (Jack fruit liquor)

(iii) *Kadali-kalu* (Plantain liquor)

(iv) *Guda-kalu* (Molasses liquor)

(v) *Mada-kalu* (*Sago*-palm juice)

(vi) *Duri-kalu* (Rice or *Ragi* liquor) and

(vii) *Amba-kalu* (Mango-liquor)[23]

The use of liquor is not socially prohibited to any sex and age. Taking liquor is a common practice and approved by the society. They get drunk to get rid of boredom and hard-labour. It is also a medicine when anybody suffers from cold and headache. *Kutia* Kondhs take four types of liquor, viz. (i) *madanga* (juice of *sago*-palm tree), (ii) *akinga* (fermented liquor made from *mahua* flower), (iii) *katuli* (fermented liquor made from one kind of millet) and (iv) *pranga ankinga* (rice-beer).[24] *Desia* Kondhs are very much addicted to drinking. Three types of liquor, viz. (i) *irpi kalu* (*mahua* liquor), (ii) *mada kalu* (*sago*-palm juice) and (iii) *kajuri kalu* (date-palm juice) are taken by them. Some herbs and roots are added to the juice to make it more intoxicating. They also take fermented liquor prepared from rice, maize and *ragi*.[25]

Drinking habit affects their lungs, kidney and liver. Cirrhosis of liver has been a common disease among them. The Kondhs feel that fresh *sago*-palm juice and *mahua* liquor have food value. Liquor is an energetic stimulant which breaks the monotony and a food which satisfies starving belly. It is a recognised means of relaxation and reducing strain. Being shifting cultivators, they undertake enough of hazardous jobs. They ransack the forest to take out their livelihood. They ascend and descend the hill-tops by going and coming from the fair-price and market centre. Liquor is one of the charming drinks for them for all such strains. But excess of it creates problem for them physically and socially.[26]

Drugs and Narcotics

Kondhs are inveterate smokers. Kondhs also use various types of narcotics and stimulants like *kara, dhongla, kundeli* and *chunga*. *Kara* is prepared out of dry and raw tobacco leaf and fine ash. Raw tobacco or *dua* is simply pressed and chewed which is known as *dhangla*. *Kundeli or topari* is otherwise known as *pika*. Tobacco leaf is rolled in *siali*-leaf and used as country made cigars. *Chunga* is tobacco container pipe used for smoking. There are two types of *chunga* or *bidi*, smaller one is used by the women and bigger one is used by the men. The amount of narcotics consumed by a person depends on his or her personal taste and capacity to offer the cost.[27] They usually keep the *dua* or raw tobacco between the lower lip and incisor teeth for sometimes and then spit out. It is taken both by male and female and they are addicted to it. All such habits are too dangerous for the health and lead to various health disorders. It affects their heart, lungs, teeth and mouth. They are aware of the adverse effects of these habits still they continue it due to tension of work-pressure or with pleasure.

Drinking Water and Sanitation

Water is a potent component of life and its quality is directly related to the efficacy of personal and community life. It is the most important aspect on which health completely depends. It is life and we can't live without it. Pure water is highly essential for our life but Kondh people have no such knowledge and they manage themselves with the water they get from their nearest surrounding. Kondh people are also not very much particular about the purity of water. There is no water in many of the Kondh villages and they drink water from the hill streams. And this water is used for multifarious purposes such as cooking; drinking, washing clothes, bathing, defection, scrubbing their cattle and also for cleaning their utensils. Buffaloes lie down in the stream water most often which makes the water impure. Besides, the stream water always carries decomposed leaves and other vegetative matters which provide appropriate milieu for the breeding of various kinds of parasites. It is for this reason that incidence of diarrhoea and dysentery, typhoid (amoebic and bacillary) and other gastric diseases are very common with these people. Occurrence of helminthic (worm) infestations, viz. Taenia solium, Taenia bovis and Ascaris lumbricoides (tape worm, round worm and hook worm) is high due to their food and impure water.[28] To eradicate water problem Government has sunk wells and tube wells in the tribal area. But the surrounding of the tube wells as well as wells are swampy, dirty and utterly unhygienic as the used water stagnates and people also throw all sorts of rubbish around them. Besides people take bath over there sometimes, housewives clean utensils, dirty linen and anal washing of children after defection around the tube wells and wells.[29] The polluted surrounding and water are said to be the main causes of number of diseases.

The tribal people living in different eco-systems face health and genetic problems of varying nature. The other important factors which attribute to poor health are lack of environmental sanitation, personal hygiene, poor living condition, improper ventilation and bodily cleanliness.

Environmental Sanitation

Environmental sanitation is extremely important for healthy living. Hence it is necessary to find out the environmental sanitation especially with regard to the mosquito and fly breeding. Environment of the Kondh villages remain polluted and dirty for a variety of reasons. The village street is littered with animal dung, household refuge, excreta of children and swamps of human and other dirty materials. There is no arrangement for disposal of household waste water. The water used for domestic purpose such as washing of utensils, cleaning of food materials, occasional washing of clothes, and bathing of children, sick and old persons is released to a pit located outside the house. It is allowed to soak into the ground or remain stagnant and become a favourable cradle for various types of parasites.

A good house not only offers protection against bad weather but also plays a great role in preventing the transmission of disease. Their hygienic problem starts from their dwelling house and the surrounding. Generally the Kondh's house is rectangular in ground plan. It consists of a spacious rectangular room, another small room (*dhapa*) at the back of the first room. The roofs are made so low as to leave a space of two feet from the ground to crawl into the house. A low roof of this type remains warm during winter but these houses are not quite fit for proper ventilation, fresh air and light which are absolutely essential for good health. They are not conscious about the need of fresh air and sun rays.[30] There are no windows and hardly any light gets into the hut. Poor ventilation and close contact with the infected members of the family are largely responsible for wide contagion.[31] There is no fowl-pan as such. A basket is kept in the back room. Goats are kept in the back *verandah.* During rainy season they are given shelter in the backside room. They are also fond of keeping pigs. The pigs stay close to the *verandah.* Cattle are tethered to the wooden posts in the cowshed which are either built any side or at the backside of the house. Pigeons are kept in a wooden crate and their place of stay lies in the space under the roof of the back verandah.[32] This shows that they have no separate settlement for the domestic animals. They live with them which have adverse effects on their health.

In general, the Kondh villages are unclean and unhygienic from various angles. The cowshed, pigsty and poultry shed are all located in the house where the family members live. Both men and animals live together in the same house under one roof. Village lanes are filthy and unclean on account of deposition of cow-dung and dried leaves here and there. The pigs which they rear make the surrounding filthier. During rainy season water accumulates on the lanes and the areas become muddy and filthy. Their dwellings are not kept clean as both the female and male members are busy in their economic activity and do not get time to clean their house. Only on festive occasion houses are cleaned and walls are plastered with clay mixed with cow-dung.[33]

They are indifferent to the unhygienic practices such as, existence of cow shed close to the house, conversion of half of *verandah* into a shed for the domestic animals like goats and sheeps, spitting anywhere such as in every corner of the house or below the *verandah* or steps in front of the house where the small children crawl. They throw the empty bottles, broken combs and unused rotten things here and there which the small children usually bite and it has a bad effect on their health. The left out food is thrown around the cemented floor of the tube-wells, non canalisation of the dirty water around the tube-well, throwing of waste products like paper, torn clothes; dry leaves etc. on the stocks create shelter for the flies and insects.[34]

Personal Hygiene

The term personal hygiene includes all those personal factors which influence the health and well being of an individual. In a broad sense it comprises a range of day to day activities such as bodily care, bathing, washing, care of clothes, hair, teeth, skin and nails, sleep, exercise, diet etc. and on the whole a systematic organised way of healthy life. Any disruption of these activities may impair health. The Kondhs lack this sense of hygiene. This causes many diseases.

Bath is not taken every day and they have no proper time for bath. During summer they take a bath whenever they like but in winter they do not bath for months together. Once they climb the hills in the morning to reach the *dongar* for working, they feel reluctant to climb down again to stream for bath. They wash their head once or twice in a month. They use one kind of soil for it. They use soap rarely. Generally they take bath in rivulet. During rainy season water of the rivulet becomes muddy and soiled. Sometimes in other seasons also it becomes muddy and soiled due to the bathing of the buffaloes. Still then they bath in rivulet, this results in causing a number of infectious diseases.

No regularity is maintained to wash teeth and face, as and when required teeth are cleaned with mango twigs. General health of teeth is very poor. Most adults show yellow teeth and suffer from disorders like caries and tartar. It is due to poor dental hygiene.[35]

Kondhs follow open air defecation. The adults get up around 5 a.m. and they go to the nearby forest for defecation. After discharge of faeces the excreta is cleaned with any green leaves readily available and water is rarely used. Ladies too do not use water after defecation or after urination. Most of the Kondhs attend natures call in open fields. They do not use soap to wash their hands.

Apart from a few well to do families soap is not used for cleaning cloths or body. *Chili-mati* is used by both men and women for cleaning hair as and when time permits. With the help of fine ash dirty clothes are cleaned with warm water and then rinsed. The ladies usually clean their clothes. Male never wash their clothes since it is considered as a female's job and hence derogatory for men. The Kondhs are not very particular in cutting the fingernails. The children often cut short the nails by biting. Their nails are often covered with dirt, which contains disease-causing micro-organisms. They may enter the body along with the food and cause illness. Nails are cut after a month or two. Hair too is not regularly cut. They cut each other's hair as there is no professional barber. If time permits oil is used on hair.[36] Males are not regular in shaving their face. Usually they shave their face once in a fortnight. Bathing in the same pond or stream along with bovine animals, non-use of water for anal washing after defecation, non-washing of hands and mouth after eating meal do have adverse impacts on health.[37]

The Kondhs predominantly wear cotton clothes but when the nights are very cold in the higher elevations they sometimes use old sweaters or some warm clothes. Kondhs are not so careful for their dresses. Small children only put on briefs and even remain naked. Some children have only one pair of clothes. They always wear that pair and hence do not wash their clothes. They use the same dress for three to four days and wash them afterwards. One person may not have more than two pairs of dress. Many people wear the same dress in the night, which they have worn while working in the field during the day time. The old folk largely use their traditional dress.

Kondhs are not careful about the cleanliness of their utensils. The cleanliness of utensils is directly related to the food hygiene. As they are economically weak, some people use their own utensils for feeding the domestic animals such as dogs, pigs, cats and mongoose. They are not careful about this important part of habit which is directly linked to their health.[38]

Usually they go to sleep around 8 p.m. shortly after taking supper. As the hamlets are situated in high elevations, surrounded by the forest, the temperature is very low at night. So they put up fire to quell cold. The Kondhs sleep on the floor. Some wealthy Kondhs use wooden cots while majority of them use a sack or a mat woven with the leaves of trees or grass. The dormitory system exists in this tribal community. The unmarried youths spend the night in separate male and female dormitories. In a dormitory they sleep very close to each other. Sick persons also sleep in the dormitory which may pave the way for the spreading of diseases. People are not aware of this problem.

Kondhs are too careless for the hygiene of their children. They are not careful about the cleanliness of the children. Children and pregnant women are completely neglected. They live in such an unhygienic condition that they suffer from many diseases.[39]

There is no change in the day to day work of women when they are pregnant. As usual they work hard even up to their delivery stage. In insanitary surrounding the delivery is made. The mother herself cuts the umbilical cord of the baby by means of bamboo strip or by a piece of broken pottery which is not hygienic. In the post natal period the mother is given rice and salt only for a few days with the belief that there would be more lactation from her breasts. The poor economic condition handicaps the Kondhs to purchase nutritious food for both the mother and child. It is found that infants in these poor families live totally on breast feeding. Mothers keep on breast feeding till the birth of second issue. As the mothers do not get nutritious food, they fail to produce more milk. As a result their milk becomes insufficient for the child. Consumption of cow milk is a taboo among them, as they believe that if the calf is deprived of cow's milk their women will not lactate and their children will be deprived of breast feeding. So they give supplementary food, which includes boiled papayas, potatoes and grains. Due to financial stringency they cannot purchase vegetables or any nutritious food. They manage themselves with the vegetables which they get from the kitchen garden and forest. Their illiteracy and negligence make their children victim of imbalance diet.

After the baby is grown up he or she is also neglected. They are left at their own risk as if they know how to care themselves. They are not careful to watch the baby for his/her daily work, such as bathing, clothing and cutting nails. Generally up to two/ three years of age mother or elder sister is concerned about brushing the teeth of the child, cutting nails, rubbing oil on hair and body, bathing etc. However they never do these timely. When the child starts walking he/she comes in contact with dirty dust, cow-dung and other nasty things and hence suffers from various infectious diseases. When the child becomes three years old, the mother or elder sister is no more careful for the personal hygiene of the child. So the children manage themselves.

Running noses is a common feature of all children below the age of eight throughout the year as they play with water near the rivulet or stream or tube-well. Utter negligence in cleaning running noses also causes wounds below the nose.[40]

These people are too careless for their health and environment. They believe that the health is ensured by supernatural entities. Factors like regular bathing, washing of clothes, cleaning of head-hair, regular washing of mouth, regular clipping of nails and toes are not considered as essential from the point of view of good health.

Diseases are constant challenge to human health and existence. Tribes consider health and disease are two polar opposites. Disease refers to departure from the state of health and health is the absence of disease. Although welfare programmes of Government has brought improvement in the lifestyle of the tribes in general and Kondhs in particular but there is no change in their attitude towards health.[41] Their health status is marked by poverty, illiteracy, malnutrition, lack of personal hygiene, poor sanitation, non availability of pure drinking water with poor maternal and child birth services. These factors affect the health status of the tribal's adversely and are also responsible for some of the specific illness including genetic disorders. Unfortunately proper health services are not available in many of the tribal areas including that of the Kondhs.

The health status of the Kondh in general is reported to be in poor condition. Their health and sickness are influenced in general by a combination of biological, cultural and environmental factors. The health of the Kondh is mostly affected by insufficient diet, lack of personal hygiene, poor sanitation facilities and various socio-cultural practices. The health problems among the Kondhs can be grouped into the following main categories.

(i) High rate of infectious and water borne diseases (diarrhoea, dysentery, skin disease).

(ii) Poor environmental sanitation and hygiene (communicable diseases like malaria, tuberculosis, venereal diseases, etc.).

(iii) Malnutrition (macro-and micronutrient deficiencies).

(iv) Genetic diseases (sickle cell disease and haemoglobinopathies).

(v) An unsatisfactory health care delivery system (public health).[42]

Malaria

Malaria is the foremost public health problem of Odisha contributing to 23 per cent of malaria cases, 40 per cent of plasmodium falciparum cases and 50 per cent of malaria deaths in the country. More than 60 per cent of the tribal population of Odisha lives in high risk areas for malaria. Though the tribal communities constitute nearly 8 per cent of the total population of the country, they contribute 25 per cent of the total malaria cases and 15 per cent of total plasmodium falciparum cases. Various

epidemiological studies and malariometric surveys carried out in tribal population, including primitive tribes, reveal a high transmission of plasmodium falciparum in the forest regions because malaria control in such settlements has always been unattainable due to technical and operational problems. A prospective study conducted by Regional Medical Research Centre (RMRC), Bhubaneswar during 2000-2003 in Malkangiri and Kandhamala districts shows that slide positivity rate (SPR) is 10.5 per cent in Kondhs. The plasmodium falciparum (PF) per cent is 92.7 in Kondhs. It is observed that these districts are endemic for malaria.

Diarrhoea Disorders

Water-borne communicable diseases like gastrointestinal disorders including acute diarrhoea are responsible for a higher morbidity and mortality among Kondhs. It is due to poor sanitation, unhygienic conditions and lack of safe drinking water in the Kondh settlement. In a cross sectional study conducted by the RMRC, Bhubaneswar, in 2003, in four primitive tribes of Odisha (Bondo, Didayi, Kondh and Juang), the diarrhoea diseases including cholera are found to occur throughout the year attaining its peak during the rainy season. During 2002-2003, 10.4 per cent of Kondh children (0-6 years) and 10.2 per cent Kondh adult population were suffering from acute diarrhoea. The acute diarrhoea problem is basically due to the poor environmental hygiene, lack of safe drinking water, improper disposal of human excreta which is further aggravated by low literacy, low socio-economic status coupled with blind cultural belief, lack of access to medical facilities leading to serious public health problem.

Intestinal Parasitism

Intestinal protozoan and helminthes infestations are the major public health problems. As per the survey report of RMRC, Bhubaneswar, 2003, 41.1 per cent of Kondh primitive tribes of Odisha were suffering from this disease. Amongst helminthic infestation hookworm is the most common disease. About 18.2 per cent of Kondhs were suffering from this disease. Children (aged between 1 and14 years) were more affected than the adults. Most of these infections are due to indiscriminate defecation in the open field, bare foot walking and lack of health awareness and hygiene.[43]

Upper Respiratory Tract Infection

After anaemia, the respiratory disease including upper respiratory tract infection is more commonly prevalent. As per the

Report of RMRC, Bhubaneswar, it was 13.6 per cent among Kondhs. This accounts for a high infant mortality due to inadequate vaccination, lack of early diagnosis and prevention.

Micronutrient Deficiency

Micronutrient deficiency is closely linked with nutritional disorders and diarrhoea. Deficiency of essential dietary components leads to malnutrition, protein calorie deficiency and micronutrient deficiencies (like vitamin A, iron and iodine deficiency). Vitamin A deficiency in the form of Bitot's spot, conjunctival xerosis and night blindness was observed and it was 6.9 per cent among Kondhs.[44]

Hereditary Haematological Disorders

Hereditary haematological disorders especially sickle cell disease, Glucose-6-Phosphate Dehydrogenise (G6PD) deficiency, haemoglobinopathies and allied haemolytic disorders are important public health problems and occur in high frequencies among different tribal groups including Kondhs and scheduled caste population. These result in a high degree of morbidity and mortality due to haemolysis in vulnerable population.

Sickle cell gene is widely prevalent among the tribal population in India. These have been investigated in over 100 tribal populations. The prevalence rate varies widely from 0.5 to 45 per cent among different tribes. There are many primitive tribes who have been identified to be in high-risk group. Majority of the tribals of Odisha have a common gene pool that is relatively unmixed with other nontribal population. High degree of inbreeding among some of the primitive tribes results in relatively high prevalence of genetically inherited diseases like sickle cell anaemia, G6PD deficiency and thalassaemia. Sickle cell gene is also prevalent among the Kondhs to a great extent. The incidence of sickle cell haemoglobin was found to be 3 per cent in case of Kondhs. The frequency of sickle cell gene is reported to be low, which was about 1.5 per cent, while G6PD deficiency was 4.8 per cent among *Kutia* Kondhs. It is high especially in hyper endemic malaria zones.

Thalassaemia also contributes significantly for the anaemia cases in the tribal population of Odisha. Studies have shown that the prevalence of thalassaemia is 2.3 per cent in *Kutia* Kondh primitive tribes.[45]

Skin Disease

The skin diseases like scabies, pediculosis, monitiasis etc. are prevalent among the Kondhs. Skin problem is a major health problem amongst the Kondhs of Odisha because of overcrowding and unhygienic living conditions as also close contacts and lack of health awareness. From the study conducted by RMRC, Bhubaneswar, it is revealed that 15 per cent of the Kutia Kondh population was affected with scabies, both infective and non-infective.

Infant and Maternal Mortality

The rates of infant, child, and maternal mortalities continue to be high among Kondhs. A large number of infants die during first year of life. The incidence is reported to be very high in *Kutia* Kondhs of Phulbani district. The underlying factors are female illiteracy, early marriages, low-birth weight, malnutrition, asphyxia, dysentery, diarrhoea, gastroenteritis, jaundice, respiratory tract infection and poor availability of maternal health services. Unhygienic methods of child delivery, complicated labour problems ineptly handled by village midwives are causing death to either mother or baby or both, or cause infection to the mother and baby. The unhygienic and primitive practices are mainly responsible for high maternal mortality. It is observed that among Kutia Kondh, the delivery is conducted by the mother herself in a half squatting position holding a rope tied down from the roof of the house. This helps her in applying pressure to deliver the child. The umbilical cord of the child is cut by means of a bamboo strip or by a broken pottery instead of sterilised blade or knife by the mother.[46]

Starting from gestation period to child birth, the mother is debarred to take certain food and leaves. When the expectant mother is not getting adequate amount of balanced diet to consume it becomes difficult on her part to feed the child from her breast. The complicated labour during delivery leads to maternal as well as child mortality. Poor nutritional status makes the child more susceptible to infection, disease, slower recovery and mortality. Due to malnutrition and unhygienic living conditions, children suffer from various diseases. The children mostly in the age group of 3-10 are the victims of various diseases. Generally, they suffer from pneumonia, measles, swelling, scabies, jaundice, fungal infection, upper respiratory tracts infection (URTI), fever, diarrhoea etc. The children suffer from various skin infection and diseases in rainy season. Running noses, cold and cough are the common diseases found in this season. In summer season they suffer from prickly heat and boils, dysentery and dehydration. During the winter season usually they suffer from suffocation, cracking of skin due to excessive cold, fever, loose motion, etc.[47]

As per the report of RMRC 2002-2003, Bhubaneswar, the infant mortality rate among the Kondhs (*Kutia*) is 128.7 per thousand. Maternal mortality among Kondhs is 11.2 per thousand female populations. The life expectancy is 50.7 among Kondhs. The crude birth rate is 21.6 and death rate is 20.9 per thousand population in Kondh tribe.[48]

Gastro-intestinal Disorders

They also suffer from gastro-intestinal disorders. Unhygienic condition of the surrounding in which they live, polluted water and the water content of graphite causes irritation in the gastro-intestinal tract resulting in gastric discomfort, abdominal pain, hyper acidity and constipation. Common gastro-intestinal disorders prevalent among the Kondhs are gastritis, colitis and dyspepsia. Heavy alcoholic drinking with insufficient diets causes this diseases.[49]

Other Health Problems of Kondhs

The disease related to respiratory system is bronchitis (acute and chronic) asthma and disease of the upper respiratory tract. Influenza, cold and cough are also there. Among other diseases they suffer from are arthritis and rheumatic disorder. Arthritis and spondylitis are common. They also suffer from loss of appetite and breathlessness.[50]

Leprosy is also there among the Kondhs. Patients affected by leprosy are more in Rayagada area. People suffering from leprosy are not segregated from their society and the disease spread widely as a result of close contact with the infected patient. The incidence of tuberculosis is also high. Semi-starvation, inferior diet and unhygienic living conditions attribute to the prevalence of tuberculosis. In a prospective study undertaken in Odisha, the incidence of tuberculosis and leprosy are found to be 0.7 per cent among Kondhs.[51]

The Kondhs have very less knowledge about sexually transmitted diseases (STD). They suffer from syphilis which is transmitted mostly through sex. The local name of disease is "*bedana roga*" meaning painful disease. The Kondhs are so much afraid of this disease that a person suspected to be suffering from this disease is prohibited to urinate in public places and is required to dig a pit for self use. His or her clothes are not used by others, even he/she is not allowed to dine in community feasts. As they know the infectious nature of this disease, they follow harsh restriction for it. The other sexually transmitted disease gonorrhoea is also prevalent among the Kondhs.[52]

They have also all types of ear, nose and throat (ENT) problems. The eye diseases like conjunctiva and cornea, cataract and glaucoma constitute more. Diseases like streptococcal throat infection otitis media and mastoiditis are there. Hyper tropic tonsil is high.[53]

Due to malnutrition the incidence of nutritional and metabolic disorders is very high. The survey was conducted by Almas Ali among *Kutia* Kondhs of Burlubaru Village, Phulabani district, in the year 1979 to assess the prevalence of malnutrition and under-nutrition. The followings are the most common deficiencies observed by him.

(i) Under nutrition:
- (a) Low weight in relation to height
- (b) Diminished skin folds
- (c) Lethargy-especially in children
- (d) Exaggerated skeletal prominence
- (e) Loss of elasticity of skin

(ii) Protein-caloric deficiency:
- (a) Oedema
- (b) Muscle wasting
- (c) Moon face etc.

(iii) Vitamin A deficiency:
- (a) Xerobis of skin
- (b) Xerobis conjunctiva
- (c) Kerato malacia
- (d) Bitot's spots

(iv) Vitamin B deficiency:
- (a) Loss of ankle jerks
- (b) Calf muscle tenderness

(v) Vitamin B_2 deficiency (Riboflovin):
- (a) Angular stomatitis
- (b) Cheilosis

(c) Magenta tongue

(d) Corneal vascularisation

(vi) Vitamin C (Ascorbic Acid) deficiency:

(a) Spongy and bleeding gums

(b) Petechaiae

(vii) Vitamin D deficiency:

(a) Active rickets in children

(b) Healed rickets in children and few adults

(c) Octomalacia in adults with local skeletal deformities

(viii) Iron deficiency:

(a) Pallor or mucous membrane (anaemic)

(b) Koilonychias[54]

Low blood pressure is common but hypertension is not there among these people. Hair loss and baldness is very rare among them. This proves that they have no care for the different tensions of life and always think for the present and they are not worried for the dark future, which helps them to be free from hypertension. They are very much careful for their hair and use of natural oil helps them to be free from baldness. It is found from the field study that they always use oil extracted from *jada* (Ricinus communis) which helps for the growth and blackness of hair. Now these people are using shampoo to wash their hair due to the influence of the non-tribals.[55]

Health problems are usually much less acute in case of *Desia* Kondhs than others and more acute in case of *Kutia* Kondhs. The Kondhs suffer from a number of diseases. These are scabies and other skin diseases, trachoma, inflammatory diseases of eye, cataract, glaucoma, otitis media and mastoiditis, Streptococcal throat infection, hyper trophic tonsil, asthma, lobar-pneumonia, bronchial-pneumonia, chronic bronchitis, acute bronchitis, tuberculosis (respiratory), URTI (upper respiratory tract infection), amoebic dysentery, bacillary dysentery, dysentery mixed, stomach ulcer, duodenal ulcer, gastritis and other digestive disorders, teeth and gum diseases, menorrhagia, abortion, arthritis, spondylitis, rheumatism muscular and related diseases, rheumatic fever, neuritis, other diseases of sense organs, avitaminosis and other deficiency diseases, pellagra, anaemia, influenza, whooping cough, leprosy, measles, typhoid, syphilis, malaria, filariasis, other helminthic diseases, diarrhoea, G6PD deficiency, thalassaemia, jaundice, heart trouble, dermatitis, conjunctivitis and eczema.[56]

These unlettered tribal people steeped in traditional practices lack an understanding of environmental sanitation and personal hygiene in the context of health and prevention of diseases. When 70.4 per cent of tribal people in the country are illiterate, half fed, ill-clothed and deprived of portable drinking water, their attitude towards environmental sanitation and personal hygiene is bound to be archaic and in tune with their traditional world view.[57]

Socio-cultural facts associated with variations in age, sex, ethnicity, occupation and community can have significant bearings on epidemiological phenomena. Age, sex and occupational differences have correlations with the incidence of certain types of diseases.

Age Differences

Due to lack of physiological resistance tribal children are susceptible to several diseases such as diarrhoea, dysentery, dyspepsia, common cold, fever, jaundice, scabies, ring worm, anaemia, etc. Death rate is relatively high among infants. The incidence of numerous acute infections is higher among children, tribal as well as non-tribal. As people grow older they develop immunities that decrease their vulnerability to diseases.

Sex Differences

Biological factors play a large part in sexual differences and mortality with females having longer life expectancy. However, women frequently suffer from reproductive diseases sustaining ovary and breast ailments. Men on the other hand are affected by renal and cardiovascular diseases. More tribal women suffer from arthritis as they are frequently anaemic and always carry heavy loads on their head. Several tribal women after child birth suffer from gynaecological and obstetric problems and in the process become vulnerable to other types of ailments.

Occupational Difference

There is a correlation between occupation and disease. Effects of occupation on disease have been an important aspect of epidemiology because social aspects of pathology indicate that susceptibility to disease varies in accordance with the means of livelihood. Tribals who rear pigs suffer from worm infection, likewise tribals working in cement factories suffer from thoracic disease.[58] Such differences are there among the Kondhs.

According to the latest report of National Nutrition Monitoring Bureau (NNMB) 2000-2001, Odisha continues to have second highest level of under nutrition among the ten states. The survey conducted by RMRC, Bhubaneswar, reported that chronic energy deficiency is found to be very high among the Kutia Kondhs (88.9 per cent) of Rayagada district. Anaemia is another problem which is more in females than males.[59]

Thus the above account reveals that the condition of health and the health consciousnesses among the Kondhs are below average. However at present the various programmes launched by Government agencies including Integrated Tribal Development Agency (ITDA) have motivated the Kondhs to realise their pitiable unsanitary condition and degradation of their standard of health. Therefore, they are gradually accepting the various health programmes for better living. Many voluntary organisations and missionaries have become active in the Kondh inhabited tribal areas for the upliftment of the health standard of Kondhs, their sanitary condition and environment for a safe and sound living. As a result of which malaria and skin diseases have been lessened considerably, child and mother death rate have been reduced significantly. It is hoped that adequate medical facilities, improved sanitary condition and health consciousness will be helpful to get cured from diseases and decrease in the mortality rate among Kondhs.

The Kondhs even today are away from the path of civilisation and lead a life of squalor, poverty and misery. Unfortunately this tribal group of Odisha has little or no access even to the most elementary and rudimentary form of health care. Paradoxically enough they are the very people who have utmost need of health care because they are most vulnerable to disease and have high degree of morbidity and malnutrition.

Good health and good society go together. This would be possible only when a number of supportive services such as improvement in environment, nutrition and education go up to a very high level. In this task special care should be taken for providing adequate health care for the Kondhs. The major health problems can be avoided by ensuring safe drinking water, curative and preventive health care, health education, etc., to Kondhs. To bring more development, the modern medical facilities should be available at their door steps.

References

1. Krishan Sharma, *The Konds of Orissa*, Concept Publishing Company, New Delhi, 1979, 34.
2. *Indian Council of Medical Research (herein after ICMR) Bulletin*, Vol. 33, No. 10, October, 2003, "Health Status of Primitive Tribes of Orissa", http:llwww.icmr.nic.in/BVOCTO3.
3. N. Patnaik, *The Kondh,* Tribal Harijan Research cum Training Institute (herein after THRTI), Bhubaneswar, 1989, 25.
4. Mohan Advani and Mohammad Akram, "Health Concerns in India" in Mohammad Akram, (ed.), *Health Dynamics and Marginalised Communities*, Rawat Publication, New Delhi, 2007, 3-5.
5. Gopinath Mohanty and Ajit Kumar Maharana, "Oleopathy, It's Use by Different Tribes", in *Adivasi*, Vol. 45, No-2, Dec. 2005, Scheduled Castes and Scheduled Tribes Research and Training Institute (hereinafter SCSTRTI), Bhubaneswar, 1.
6. Almas Ali, "Health Status of Tribals in India: An overview", in Dipak Kumar Adak, Biswanath Bhattacharya, Rohini Ghosh, Manoranjan Pal, Premananda Bharati and T. S. Vasulu (eds.), *Demography and Health Profile of the Tribals*, Anmol Publication, 2003, 1-2.
7. *ICMR Bulletin, op. cit.*
8. Pratap Kumar Singh, "Health Hazards on Tribal Societies of Orissa and It's Remedy" in Jyotsna Mohany (ed.), *Tribal Health, Culture and Development in Orissa*, Kamla Nehru College, Bhubaneswar, 2004, 178-179.
9. Krishan Sharma, *op.cit.*, 42.
10. *The Kandha of Orissa*, SCSTRTI, 2006, 23-26.
11. S.K. Basu and A. Jindal, *A Report on "Genetic and Socio-Cultural Dimensions of Tribal Health – A Primitive Kutia Kondh of Phulabani District"*. Unpublished Report., ICMR Project, New Delhi, 1990, 28.
12. *The Kandha of Orissa*, SCSTRTI, 2006, 315.
13. Pratap Kumar Singh, *op.cit.,* 179.
14. L.S.S. O'Malley, *Bengal District Gazetteers, Angul,* Calcutta, 1908, 67-68.
15. *The Kandha of Orissa*, SCSTRTI, *op. cit.*, 55-56.
16. Mihir Kumar Jena, Padmini Pathi, Kamala Kumari Patnaik and Klaus Seeland, *Forest Tribes of Orissa,* Vol. 2, *Kuttia Kondh*, D.K. Print World, New Delhi, 2006, 81.

17. Krishan Sharma, *op.cit.*, 39-40.

18. Sujata Senapati, "Health Nutrition and Genetic Problems of the Tribal Communities in Orissa" in Jyotsna Mohanty, (ed,), Tribal Health, Culture and Development in Orissa, Kamla Nehru College, Bhubaneswar, 2004, 184.

19. *The Kandha of Orissa*, SCSTRTI, *op. cit.*, 397.

20. Krishan Sharma, *op. cit.*, 44.

21. *The Kandha of Orissa*, SCSTRTI, *op. cit.*, 24.

22. N.K. Behura and K.K. Mohanti, *Tribal Orissa, Reading in Social Anthropology*, Dominant Publisher, New Delhi, 2006, 115.

23. P.S. Das Pattnaik, "Liquor Among the Dongria Kondh of Orissa", in *Adivasi,* Vol. XVI, No. 3, October, 1976, SCSTRTI, Bhubaneswar, 52-53.

24. *The Kandha of Orissa*, SCSTRTI, *op. cit.*, 294.

25. *Ibid.*, 315-316.

26. P.S. Das Pattnaik, *op. cit.*, 56.

27. *The Kandha of Orissa*, SCSTRTI, *op. cit.*, 29.

28. *Ibid.*, 393.

29. N.K. Behura and K.K. Mohanti, *op. cit.*, 108.

30. *The Kandha of Orissa*, SCSTRTI, *op. cit.*, 11.

31. Almas Ali, "*Health and Genetic Problems of Kutia Kondh of Burlubaru Village, Phulabani District, Orissa.*" Unpublished Report, SCSTRTI, Government of Orissa, 1979, 5.

32. *The Kandha of Orissa*, SCSTRTI, *op. cit.*, 12-13.

33. *Ibid.*, 209.

34. Nibedita Nath, "Reproductive and Child Health Among the Kondh: Data From the District of Rayagada, in Orissa", in Jyotsna Mohanty (ed.), *Tribal Health, Culture and Development in Orissa*, Kamla Nehru College, Bhubaneswar, 2004, 161.

35. Krishan Sharma, *op. cit.*, 46.

36. Nibedita Nath, *op. cit.*, 161-162.

37. N.K. Behura and K.K. Mohanti, *op. cit.*, 115.

38. *Ibid.*, 116.

39. Nibedita Nath, *op. cit.*, 155.

40. *Ibid.*, 161-162.

41. R.K. Kar, "Ethnomedicine and Tribal Health; An Illustrative Appraisal" in A.K. Kalla, P.C. Joshi (ed.), *Tribal Health and*

Medicines, Concept Publishing Company, New Delhi, 2004, 381.

42. G. Bulliyya, *et al.*, "Indigenous Health Care Practices among the Kondh Tribal Communities of Orissa, India" in Awadesh N. Sharma, *et al.*, (eds.), *Indigenous Health Care and Ethnomedicine*, Sarup and Sons, New Delhi, 2006, 59.
43. *ICMR Bulletin, op.cit.*
44. P.K. Mohanty, *Encyclopedia of Scheduled Tribes in India*, Vol. 4, Isha Books, Delhi, 2006, 162-164.
45. *Ibid.*, 165-167.
46. *ICMR Bulletin, op. cit.*
47. Nibedita Nath, *op. cit.,*158.
48. *ICMR Bulletin, op. cit.*
49. N. Patnaik, *op. cit.,* 25-26.
50. *The Kandha of Orissa*, SCSTRTI, *op. cit.,* 394.
51. *ICMR Bulletin, op. cit.*
52. Saraswati Swain, *"Study on Health and Morbidity Status of the Tribal Population of Orissa with Special Reference to S.T.D."* sponsored by ICMR, New Delhi, 1988, Unpublished Report, 37.
53. Krishan Sharma, *op. cit.,* 29.
54. Almas Ali, *"Health and Genetic Problems of Kutia Kondh of Burlubaru Village, Phulabani District, Orissa."* Unpublished Report SCSTRTI, Government of Orissa, 1979, 7-8.
55. Personal communication during fieldwork with Sahadev Dehuri (Medicine man), Jamujhari, Khajuripada, Kandhamal, on 24.05.2010.
56. Krishan Sharma, *op. cit.,* 28-29.
57. N.K. Behura and K.K. Mohanti, *op. cit.,* 109.
58. *Ibid.,* 115-116.
59. P.K. Mohanty, *op. cit.,* 159-160.

3

Beliefs and Practices

Religion is a belief in the existence of supernatural forces which are beyond the control of man. For the tribals religion plays an important role in all spheres of their lives. Even in health care, religious beliefs and practices have their own specific influences. Because of the lack of proper health education, they derive the causes of many of their diseases from religious teachings. Thus the supernatural forces play a direct role in the causation and cure of many of the diseases. The medicine man of the community acts as mediator between the people and the supernatural power. They make offerings to the deities and ancestral spirits on behalf of the patients. They believe that a cordial relationship with the deities and ancestral spirit will ensure good health for the members of the community. So they perform various ceremonies. They believe that if a proper propitiation is not offered to the deities and ancestors then they will get angry and send disease and calamities to the members of the community.[1] It is obvious that religion is concerned with the system of beliefs, system of relationships and actions.

The religious foundation of any community has two inter-related constituents viz., beliefs and practices. Beliefs are characters for rituals. Practices are followed according to belief system. Belief is the mode of conception and practices are the mode of action. These are the starting points of major actions of a society.

The body of beliefs and concepts existing in a society with regard to the nature, origin and treatment of diseases is found always integrated with the other institutions and organisations of the society. Religious beliefs, moral codes, social values etc. had influenced the beliefs and practices of aetiology of illness and treatment in primitive societies. Cultural patterns and religious beliefs, economy and morality, social values and medical beliefs are all found together to form the health culture of a community.[2] Not only the tribal culture is varied and fascinating but also a lot of variations are observed in their concept of health, disease, treatment, life and death. Accordingly the tribal society is guided by traditionally laid down customs and every member of the society is expected to confirm it. The fate of an individual and the community at large depends on their relationship with unseen forces which interferes with human affairs. If men offend them, the mystical power punishes them by sickness, death and other natural calamities. Disease is caused by bad spirits. Spirits become bad when one has not properly propitiated them. Thus to a tribal mind, the real enemies of human health and prosperity are the gods and dead.[3] Every culture has its own beliefs and practices concerning diseases. The relationship with the gods, goddesses and ancestral spirits play a decisive role in the occurrence of diseases in the society. A harmonic relationship with the supernaturals often ensures protection from diseases and other calamities.[4]

Tribes including Kondhs believe that their life and work is controlled by supernatural beings whose abode is around them in hills, forests, rivers and houses. It is very difficult to standardise gods and spirits as their composition continually change when old ones are forgotten with the introduction of the new ones. Their gods differ from one another in composition, function and nature. They believe that diseases are caused by sprits. Some are benevolent, some are neutral and some are malevolent. The malevolent spirits and gods are cared more than their benevolent counterparts as they can bring misery. Kondhs worship a number of gods and goddesses for the eradication of disease and for a better life.

Dharani Penu

At the top of the gods and goddesses stands *Dharani Penu* (Earth Goddess), the Supreme Goddess. She is respected with high esteem as the creator of the world and does not ordinarily cause any harm to men. She protects them from pestilence, depravity and evil. She is all powerful and highest of all deities. She is therefore worshipped in all ceremonies as a mark of honour and respect. All rituals start with the name of *Dharani Penu*. She is usually satisfied by human blood. She is responsible for growth, vegetation and product of land. She is installed in a hut in the front yard of each village called *Kudeli*. In addition to her, the village deity *Jatrakudi is* also installed there.

Kotebadi Penu

Next to *Dharani Penu*, a male deity is worshipped called *Kotebedi Penu* who is believed to be the husband of *Dharani Penu*. He is supposed to keep constant watch over the village and protect Kondhs from any mishap. He is worshipped, whenever *Dharani Penu* is worshipped on any occasion.

Other than *Dharani Penu* and *Kotebadi Penu*, they worship number of gods and goddesses and propitiate them through appropriate rites, sacrifices, charms and spells. Kondhs do not build any temple for their deities, only block of stones are erected in different places outside the village for the purpose of worship.

Takarani Penu

Next to *Dharani Penu* and *Kotebadi Penu* Kondhs worship *Takrani Penu*. She is an important female deity. She is supposed to reside at one end of the village and is responsible for the occurrence of small pox, cholera, infectious diseases, accidents and animal related diseases. She is worshipped with elaborate rituals and sacrifices. The individual who suffers from diseases usually makes votive offerings to her.

Hira Penu

Hira Penu is a female deity considered to be the maid servant of *Takrani Penu*. She inflicts pain on the children if not properly worshipped.

Chatar Penu

Chatar Penu is a male spirit who is represented by a post (*munda*). He is worshipped by *Bejuni* inside the house during *meriah* festival. He is very pernicious in bringing diseases if not properly appeased. To please him Kondhs sacrifice buffalo.

Banjari Penu

He is considered very powerful like *Chatar Penu* and is represented by a (*munda*) post and is appeased with the sacrifice of a cow to avert epidemics in the village.

Bhairo Penu

Bhairo Penu is a male spirit and brings accidental deaths in the family, if not appeased with a major sacrifice like cow.[5]

Soru Penu

Soru Penu is a female spirit and is directly related to *Dharani Penu*. This goddess stays in the hills and is worshipped just before the first clearing of hills for shifting cultivation. It is believed that a person who is in search of medicinal plants on the hill must offer prayer to this *Penu*. Particular herbs like *raga mara* and *bichu mara* are reputed to save lives and can only be gathered by a person who has received orders from *Soru Penu* in a dream. It is believed that these special herbs will be instantly vanished if some unauthorised person attempts to collect them.[6]

Piju Penu

The *Piju Penu* is a male deity who resides in the nearby stream of the village. This deity has no image or shrine. The ritual is conducted before *Piju Penu* by the *jani*. He worships this deity to cure the illness of the family members.

Jaka Penu

This deity is a male god and resides on the roof of every Kutia Kondh house but is not represented by any object or image. This god is worshiped for the fulfilment of any vow made by the head of the household to cure diseases of the family members. The ritual of this deity is performed by the *kutaka*. A goat/hen/pigeon is sacrificed to appease this deity.

Kuti Penu

This goddess resides near the stream and does not have any image or shrine. She is worshipped for joint and waist pain. The *jani* forecasts to the diseased person in which stream the particular *Kuti Penu* resides who has administered the disease. Then the *jani* accompanies the diseased person to the particular stream and performs ritual. A pig is sacrificed for that purpose.

Baburai Penu

This goddess resides inside the house of Kutia Kondh and is worshipped by the *kutaka* on the occasion of *Badabiha Dakina* festival for health, production and betterment of the family.

Linga Penu and Janan Penu

Linga Penu and *Janan Penu* stay together. These deities reside inside every Kutia Kondh's house. Kutia Kondh believes that *Linga Penu* and *Janan Penu* reside over the departed soul and is responsible for the disease of pregnant woman and the new born. To cure the diseases rituals are performed with pig/goat/chicken/pigeon sacrifice. The *kutaka* performs these rituals.

Timba Dedi

She is a family goddess and is worshipped by the *kutaka* to cure a person from fever. Only chicken is sacrificed to appease this deity.[7]

Jugah Penu

Jugah Penu is the god of small-pox. She is worshipped on all possible occasions as *Thakurani*. They use to say that *Jugah Penu* sows small-pox upon mankind as a man sows seeds upon the earth. When a village is threatened with this dreadful disease, it is deserted by all except a few who remain to offer the blood of buffaloes, dogs and sheeps to the destroying power. The inhabitants of the neighbouring hamlets try to prevent its approach by planting thorns along their paths which led towards the infected places.[8]

Gari Penu

Gari Penu is worshiped when the birth of a child does not take place in proper time. Then the priest takes the lady to the confluence of two streams, sprinkle water over her and makes an offering to the deity. When any animal becomes devoid of fertility the same god is invoked.[9]

Niyamraja Penu

He is represented by a sword worshipped during *Dussehera* and *Jura parab*. He is supposed to save the people from unnatural death and accidents. This deity does not have any permanent abode in the village. The Dongrias call him as their first ancestor. He is said to have direct communication with Sun God (*Gama Penu*). He rules over the Niyamgiri hill under the direction of Sun God. Although they believe *Niyamraja Penu* as their ancestor they never consider him as a *duma*, rather he is propitiated as god. The name *Niyamraja* is related to his role as law maker, as directed by *dhrama devata*. He punishes those who undertake mass hunting in the forest or clear forest patches without appeasing him. When a mishap occurs in the forest *Niyamraja's* help is sought.

Gangi Penu

She is the deity of stream water sources and her abode is believed to be on high hills, particularly at the source of springs. She is known to cause diseases as punishment and is therefore worshipped in the hope of cure. When she appears in a dream as a woman carrying an earthen pot to the left, on her waist, she is thought to be communicating her indication to help. A large cigar in the right-hand indicates impending violence.[10]

Sandi Penu

She is the deity of the village boundary which marks the conjunction of the village with the forest. Her overall responsibility is to protect people from outside influence, witches or spirits. She is worshipped during the conduct of death rite. Her most important task is to ward off evil minded people, wizards, witches and spirits from entering into the village. She is believed to be ever helpful towards the people. She causes no harm to her people but violence to the evil spirits from outside, causing epidemic.

Turkee Penu

Turkee Penu resides at the village entrance. Every village has its own *Turkee Penu*. She is invoked, aimed at driving away evil spirits as she is responsible for finding off intruders. It is believed that disease can only enter the village after being permitted by *Turkee Penu* to pass.[11]

Ilu Penu

Ilu Penu is the home deity of Kondhs. Every Kondh home has *Ilu Penu*. She is responsible for the well-being of the family in general, protecting the health of each member of the family from disease, danger and to ward off evil spirits in particular. She promotes the prosperity of the house if she is appeased properly. There is an emotional bond between people and their home. The home is the centre of the family life and it is believed that home itself is a god or goddess. *Ilu* is a *Kui* word for house. The home deity *Ilu Penu* is regarded as the family deity is represented either by a single wooden post or by three wooden posts made from *sal* tree. Each post is simply decorated with carved rings..[12]

Kidi Penu

The abode of *Kidi Penu* is believed to be in large trees near a paddy field or water reservoir. Fever is seen as a punishment for disregarding the deity. They believe that the fever will cease if the deity's wishes are fulfilled. She is also appeased before crop reaping. It is believed that a crop reaped before appeasement causes the deity to continue to dwell within the grains and that the ingestion of grain leads to health disorders.

Kadiya Penu

She is worshipped to get cured from water-borne diseases and some other related pains. The rite is held in the river. She is appeased by the priest with some offerings like pork.[13]

Deu Kudu Penu and Satari Penu

These two are placed either together or separately in small thatched huts made for them beneath a large tree. These deities safeguard the welfare of the villagers and the village settlement by warding off evil spirits and in particular the spirits responsible for epidemic.

Kamati or Kamatali Penu, Manali Penu and Mardi Penu

These are three malevolent sister deities feared by the Kutia Kondh. They are believed to cause small pox, stomach disease and blood vomiting. These deities are worshipped under banyan tree.[14] *Kamati Penu* is comparable to Devi Durga. Kondhs invoke this goddess to get rid of small-pox. She is malevolent.[15]

Kondhs believe that disease is influenced by their relationship with the environment and by the supernatural powers rather than on the basis of physiological evidences. According to them disease is something that affects body and soul. It manifests itself as a physical problem in a part of the body, while sensation of pain weakens the victim physiologically. They believe that their life force or soul known as *jella* has been disturbed by some unseen power (god, goddess or spirit), which in turn causes problems throughout the body. They distinguish the physical and psychological disease. Physical disease includes dermatitis, accidental injuries, pathogenic illness, fever, diarrhoea, leprosy and other physical ailments that result from food and exposure to the environment. But the psychological illness includes fear, anxiety, epilepsy, hysteria said to be caused chiefly by evil spirit, supernatural powers and witchcraft which cannot be cured. So they have different deities, spirits believed to be identified with different diseases. They believe that the diseases which are caused due to wrath of god or spirits are called spiritual diseases. Small pox, chicken pox, measles are caused by *Kamati Penu*. Blindness, physical disorder or handicaps are called spiritual diseases.

But the natural diseases are scabies (*sengu*), eczema and ring worm (*dadu*) and vomiting (*sechkanti*), caused by the insanitary conditions of the village and therefore believed to occur naturally. Contaminated water causes diarrhoea (*patadae*), blood dysentery (*neripata*), ascariasis (*danginpdika*), amoebic dysentery (*pataklipangane*), malaria (*brapa nemberi*), fever (*nemberi*) and rhinitis (*mungu giri eju*). Cold, headache and stomach ache are believed to be caused by prolonged exposure to the environment (*aku saritei*) particularly to woods, air, sun and water. Nutritional deficiency diseases also come under this category. They consider it as poverty disease and they accept that their low economic status is responsible for their poor health.[16]

The amazing conglomeration of traditions, beliefs, sorrows and philosophies that together constitute and vitalise the rituals and festivals of the tribal's has descended from antiquity and has been preserved unimpaired to the present day. Every facet of their life covering round the year activities is intimately connected with religious beliefs and practices. These aspects of the Kondh culture give meaning and depth to their lives and solidarity to their social structure. Even if they receive instructions and orders from their gods and ancestors in their dream, they believe on their dream locally termed as *Hapna*.

Ordinarily dreams are interpreted either as good or bad. Site-seeing, talking with god, officials, making transaction in shop brings cash to the person concerned. A person suffers, if he dreams of visiting forest, climbing hill, sleeping in a cave and taking bath in the stream. It is believed that the spirit residing in the above mentioned places may like to harm the person concerned. To avoid any suffering the person concerned stops going to such places at least for a day. Dreaming like eating of ceremonial food, sweet meals bring good health for the person concerned. If died person appears in the dream, it is considered to bring economic prosperity to the family.[17]

Wild and domestic animals that appear in dreams are said to be either auspicious or inauspicious signs of impending social events. Similarly the appearance of certain type of people in dreams is said to determine the success or failure of a hunting expedition. Dreaming of a maid for example indicates the availability of at least one beast during the hunt, while dreaming a pregnant woman will lead to failure of heart. Dreaming a cow which is a symbol of goddess *Laxmi* indicates of a good harvest. If the animal in a dream seen as trapped or being killed, it signifies the livelihood of a family member being struck down by an incurable disease. Deer with whitish patches seen in a dream indicates leprosy. Dreaming a jackal is very inauspicious. A peahen standing in front of a house in the dream signifies that someone in the family will suffer an attack of epilepsy. The sight of peacock on the way to any work indicates some failure. The buffalo (*poda*) in a dream indicate a never-ending conflict between husband and wife. Cutting up a cow or bullock or buffalo represents to death of a person in the family and cutting up of one's own pet dog or pig in the dream indicates the death of somebody. Dreaming of a feast also indicates the death of a family member.[18]

They relate their dreams to some of the events to happen in the near future. Some of the diseases are believed to have happened due to the dreams seen in the last night. They have strong belief in the significance of dreams. Hence they co-relate dream with disease. The presence of certain animals and plants in dream are omens of particular disease. Some of the dreams and related consequences/diseases are mentioned below.

Interpretation of Dreams

Dreams	*Possible consequences*
A cucumber being cut	Death, abortion
A jackfruit being cut	Death, abortion
A jack fruit on tree	Birth of a son
Pumpkin in the garden	Birth of a daughter
Cucumber in the garden	Birth of a son
Eating mango	Severe coughing
Mango on tree	Mild coughing
Eating jackfruit or cucumber	Death of son or daughter

Contd...

Dreams	*Possible Consequences*
Eating pineapple	Cold, cough
Mango, pineapple, jackfruit being cut	Short life
Drinking *sago* toddy	Long life
Chilly	Eye problem
Eating orange	Coughing
Drinking liquor	Coughing
Sun	Knowledge of medicine
Death of a person	Long life
Cow	Ancestral spirit causes fever
Slashing of a cow	A good person will die by bloodshed; Violence, fever or fatal disease
Goat sacrifice	Death or fatal disease
Pigeon	Long life
Pigeon or fowl being sacrificed	*Jamarani* will decide upon life or death of a person.
Hen and chicken	Conception and easy delivery.
A girl going to take bath	Small-pox
A child floating on water	*Jugah Penu* (Small pox deity) would kill a child.
A child rescued from drowning	*Jugah Penu* (small pox deity) would spare the life of a child
New cloth	Long life.[19]

Kondh follow certain rituals and taboo during birth and death. They have a strong faith that birth and death occur due to the wish of their gods and spirits. Deference, conciliation, propitiation and submission along with animal sacrifices are the various means adopted by the Kondhs to appease the supernatural powers. The materials and objects required to satisfy the forces include unboiled rice, *sal* resin, turmeric powder, sacrifice of buffalo, cow, pig, sheep, goat, fowl or pigeon as per the necessity or demand of the deities. Animals are tortured and killed to get the desired result quickly. Eggs are also offered as ritual food to satisfy ghosts and spirits.

Birth is an occasion of rejoice for Kondhs. They have a faith that it is a moment when an ancestor gets back to life. It is believed by the Kondhs that an embryo in the mother's womb does not have a life of its own. It gets life at the moment when it is delivered. It is also believed that life comes to a child with great difficulties. It is *Jamarani* (goddess of life and death), who is the precursor of life, puts human body made up of clay (*linga*) inside the mother's womb which then grows to a child.

If problem arises at the time of delivery, it is believed that a child's life is confronted with several spirits and deities. When life (*Jiu*) comes from *Jamarani* its path is blocked by *Jugah Penu* (Small pox deity), Lada Penu, *Dharma Sania* (deity responsible for ill luck) and *Thakurani Penu* (village goddess) successively. They do not allow life to enter into the born child due to which the mother experiences labour pain for a long time. At that time the family members promise to offer ritual sacrifices. If they fail, the deities may harm the child by inflicting it with his or her characteristics i.e., the small pox deity may cause small pox, *Lada Penu* may not give right medicine to the *disari* for the treatment of the child and may cause accidental premature death. *Dharma Sania* would cause chronic diseases, *Sandi Penu* would allow malevolent spirit to create malfunctions in the child's body and *Thakurani Penu* may cause cholera epidemic. Thus a new life is always at the mercy of supernatural powers.[20]

As far as child care is concerned no special attention is paid during weaning and infancy, curious beliefs in religious fervours are prevalent regarding protecting child from the illness, injuries and accidents. Various types of beads, wood pieces and even the nails of animals are worn around the neck of the children. The most valuable and potent among these is supposed to be nail of a lion or tiger and it is considered to be the most powerful protection of children against diseases. They believe that it helps their children growing strong, free from disease and sickness. The Kondh children wear amulets and put on eye shoots (*kaji*) to escape from evil eye. The elderly male uses not only knife, bill-hook and an axe for adornment but also to escape from evil eyes. The ladies too use knife and amulets (*tabala*). Similarly there are food taboos, totemic taboos, and maturity taboos, which are observed strictly to avoid mishap.[21]

Death

Death is known as *hate* by Kondhs. They follow certain principle related to death. They observe the pollution period after death. It is believed that life and death (*jarman* or *jurma*) are determined by the Supreme Being *'Dharani Penu'* who has created this world. They accept that after death the soul goes out of the body. It turns into a spirit (*duma*) and goes away from the earth. It is always feared that death is the work of the malicious spirit, black magic or the wrath of the gods and deities. The truth is that death is unavoidable and no one can escape from this in this mortal world. It is not unknown to the Kondh, yet they cannot face this incidence of death boldly. They fight tooth and nail to save a person till his/her last gasp by administering their folk medicines and by performing all sorts of magico-religious rites. Not with standing all their efforts, if death occurs, the Kondhs console themselves and make arrangements for proper disposal of the dead. Because the soul (*Ukodi*), which activates a person to grow, rests at heaven (*Petpur*) after death and this must be satisfied as per existing norms in the society.[22]

When a pregnant woman dies the foetus is taken out of the womb and is given a separate burial because the pregnant woman is universally believed to become dangerous ghost which tries to snatch away the baby out of her womb due to frustration. In order to pin her down her bones are broken, thorns and other inhabiting materials are put in her grave where she is buried.[23] When the woman becomes ill during this period the *kutaka* is called for treatment. They believe that the illness is due to some evil spirit (*duma*) and the worship of *kutaka* will appease the evil spirit and the pregnancy can be saved. The delivery is taken place in the *jaka* (a separate enclosure) in the house in the presence of one or two experienced women. She is given some herbal medicine for easy delivery. When the baby takes birth usually the mother herself cuts the umbilical cord by means of an arrow in case of a male child but in case of a female child she cuts the cord by scythe. The mother carries the placenta and buries in the hole which is already dug by her husband on the backyard of the house and place that arrow on the spot till the remaining portion of the umbilical cord is detached from the naval of the child. If the mother falls sick immediately after the delivery then all such work is finished by some other old woman. If the child is born dead then dead body and the placenta are buried together at the outskirt of the village. The dead child and the placenta are carried by the mother herself and she places everything in the pit dug by her husband. The husband fills the pit with earth. Sometimes the *kutaka* is consulted to appease the evil spirit (*duma*). If the child bears a black spot on the left side of the body, they believe that it is good sign. If the distinct mark is seen on the right side then the *kutaka* is consulted to drive out the bad omen by performing some rituals before the *Linga Penu* at the nearby stream.

Abortion is known as *pitatuste*. It is not taken seriously by the Kondhs but some people believe that it is caused by spirit (*duma*) and they consult the *kutaka* to appease *Linga Penu*. They take herbal medicine from the *kutaka* for treatment.[24]

In case of death due to accident or premature death, a ritual is performed by the Kondhs to drive away the spirit responsible for it. Importance is given to sacrifice the cattle. Death due to witch attack is indicated with symptoms like red eyes, writhing of limbs and losing one neck bone just before the death. The priest is called to the site of worship and told to go anywhere it likes. Its movement is carefully observed by the shaman. The shaman orders a person with a gun to fire at the spirit to raise fear in the spirits mind, which ensures that the spirit will never return. Such spirits are extremely malevolent. The performance is therefore organised outside the village with gun fire. The soul after death is preserved by *Jamarani* and again sent back to the world through new birth. A person who has a normal death, there is possibility of getting a quick birth. There are restrictions for the cremation of people who die of certain diseases like leprosy (*kane*), smallpox and cholera. They are cremated at a place outside the community cremation ground. Women who die during pregnancy or children up to five years of age are cremated at a place called *ekla mahane* or *kata mahane*. Such spirits are believed to be mostly malevolent in nature.[25]

Other than the methods applied to appease the divine powers some protective measures are also adopted to escape from fear and anxiety. Kondhs specially believe in many taboos.

Taboo

The regularisation of human behaviour patronising culturally to suit the outer environment has given birth to the institution of taboo or prohibition. Kondhs regard taboo as 'holy dead', an objectified fear of the demoniac power thought to be concealed in the tabooed object. Taboo is the ritual operation intended to protect religious persons and places of worship and it prevents irreligious practices. It is believed by the Kondhs that when taboo is violated it might result in disaster.

These are productive, protective and prohibitive. They believe that unless they are prohibited from doing certain things, dreadful adversity may fall on them. Taboos associated with the process of cultivation are designed to be productive. Those like keeping women and children away from certain places, actions and objects are protective. A priest, a chief, a magician, a menstruating woman or a pregnant lady is prohibited to do certain things. If they do not obey the taboos misfortune will come to them. During menstrual period a girl is subjected to several taboos and restrictions. She should not move outside and not take any non-vegetarian or spicy and oily food. A pregnant woman is prohibited to take liquor in any form. She is forbidden from taking flesh of wild animals. She is not allowed to take pork as well as fruits like jackfruit and pumpkin. Kondhs believe that milking cow make suffer to calf and that in turn causes ill health to their children. Lactating mother is not permitted to take dry fish, fish, fibrous and nuts.[26] A pregnant women is required to follow certain taboos such as:

(i) She should not look the sun or moon during eclipse. If she looks, the child will be physically deformed.

(ii) She must not visit the burial ground which may harm the child in the womb.

(iii) She must not go to secluded places in the evening or nights so as to avoid coming under the influence of evil spirits.

(iv) In her advanced stage, she is advised to avoid heavy work because they believe it may lead to abortion or miscarriage.

Mother of the newly born child is not given any solid food on the day of delivery. Up to 21 days she is not given *ragi*-gruel, but instead, is given boiled rice and vegetable curry. She does not allow eating any green leaves as it may irritate her stomach. No salt is given to her during this period. A pinch of turmeric powder is added to the curry only. After 21 days she is given usual diet.[27]

Some food taboos are there for the pregnant lady in the Kondh community.

(i) Consumption of onion and garlic may encourage the spirits to enter the womb and the child would suffer from rash.

(ii) Consumption of fried grain is prohibited. The slimy portion of grain gets stuck to the body of the child and adversely affects its health.

(iii) Eating of *Rohu* fish (a special type of fish) causes ulcer in the umbilical region of the child, who might also suffer from rashes.

(iv) Child would suffer from tuberculosis, if boar meat is taken.

(v) Child suffers from various diseases if mother takes puffed rice during pregnancy.[28]

Other Taboos

They believe that any fruit or vegetable, if fallen on the ground, is meant for regeneration of plant and therefore not to be eaten. In this case, it is offered to any neighbour, the later can eat after touching it in his left leg. It is believed that touches with the left leg makes it free from evil influence and consequently becomes edible. Women are not allowed to eat meat of animal which are sacrificed to propitiate deities on public festive or ritual occasion. It is believed that spirits of other clan will cause harm to them.[29] After harvest the crops are first offered to the god. Pregnant women have to follow some other social restrictions. If she sees a snake by accident, she is convinced that an evil spirit dangerous to the unborn child has now entered her. To exorcise it she runs to the medicine man. The medicine man attempts to remove the evil spirit either by using an arrow as if it is a tube to suck out the evil spirit from her womb or by direct means. He expectorates into a leaf bowl and shows this to all those present explaining that he has removed the evil spirit. The bowl is then taken away to a distant place and burnt.[30]

Magic and Sorcery

Kondhs are firm believers of magic and sorcery. Certain painful experiences in their day to day life like diseases and deaths lead them to believe in the existence of an invisible spirit. It is believed that the spirit can be appeased by the chanting of some formulas which amount to the practice of some techniques for canalising the power for good and evil. This practice is called magic or sorcery. In times of sickness, the sorcerer wraps a piece of thread to which he has knotted a hair from his own head round the wrist or neck of the patient. It is removed when the patient gets completely cured. Witchcraft is universally believed by the Kondh. The Kondh has a strong belief that exercise of this art enables witches to transform themselves into tigers, leopards, wolves and so on and in this shape they attack human beings or their cattle. They believe that witches have the faculty of transferring themselves into tigers and then called *Pulto Bagho*. Kondhs believe that the witches and devils roam mainly at night time. They think that their country is full of magical beliefs and were influenced by magical notions. Hence there is no distinction between magic and religion in their eyes. They are great believers of magico-religious practices.[31] From cradle to the grave tribal man feels surrounded by evil spirits of various kinds. He offers sacrifice to appease them. Fear not devotion is the basis of his worship. The transfer of sickness from one person to another can be made through magic. Some socio-cultural superstitions, taboos, totems and evil eyes also result in the causation of few diseases. On the festive occasion the Kondhs worship many deities at different periods of life cycle.

Duma or spirit may be either benevolent or malevolent. They may extend their help in agriculture and the well being of the people. When displeased, they may also cause illness and ruin the people's well being. Apart from the spirit, the Dongria Kondhs believe in ghosts, *mahane* (unsatisfied spirits) who are controlled by shamans. They strongly believe on magical practice which is applied for both the benevolent and malevolent purposes. Therefore people depend on specialists who are expert in magical practices.[32]

Beliefs

Kondhs also believe in many more things related to life. They feel uneasy and guilty when ever certain taboo is broken and immediately they want to appease god or spirit to eradicate something wrong committed as a result of the violation of taboos.

The faith of the tribal life finds expression in tribal tradition and practices. It is through this, their strong faith on their customs and traditions are visualised. The religion of the tribal community is the result of traditions and beliefs that has come down to them from antiquity. They believe certain things without calculating the adverse result which in turn has bad effects on their body. Kondhs believe that pregnant mothers are expected to restrict their diet in quantity as there is a common fear that if the baby is too large, delivery would be difficult and might lead to death of the mother. They also restrict in terms of quality. Protein rich food is not permitted. This cultural taboo results in greater malnutrition and anemia.[33]

Their life-style, dietary pattern, social behaviour as well as health behaviour are prescribed by the deep rooted traditions that are more pronounced amongst Kondhs, where the outside influence and urbanisation are minimal. Their indigenous practices lead to more mortality rate. They assert that most diseases are caused by supernatural beings. They feel that there are five causes of sickness. These are viz. (i) displeasure of supernatural entities, (ii) breach of taboos, (iii) non- fulfilment of obligations towards manes, (iv) influence of occultism and (v) environmental and physical ones. They follow certain restrictions as per their knowledge. They do not give fibrous and hot foods to the patient who is suffering from stomach pain. *Sago* palm juice, rice-water and certain fruits (banana, custard apple) are not given to the patient who is suffering from fever and cold. Some of the taboos followed by them are more healer-oriented than patient oriented in nature.[34]

Kondhs believe deities create disease and one has to appease their deities by human and animal sacrifice. When cholera breaks out in a village all males and females smear their bodies from head to foot with pig's fat, liquefied by heat and continue to do so even few days after the disappearance of this dreadful disease. During this time they do not bath, lest the smell of the fat will be washed away. When a Kondh has an attack of fever caused by evil spirit, a ceremony is performed under a tree. They draw the circles of saffron, turmeric, charcoal, rice and some yellow powder. An egg or a small chicken is offered to the evil spirit. Kondhs are used to make attempts to keep small pox away by placing thorns and bush wood in the paths leading to places affected by the disease. They do this with a hope that the demon of the disease might retrace its steps. Usually in case of sickness the shaman or medicine man is summoned He finds the cause of the disaster and prescribes the remedy which is mostly an animal sacrifice along with offerings of grain and liquor.[35] A peculiar cultural practice among the Kondhs is that when a person is suffering from malaria or high fever and running elevated temperature, he/she is exposed to direct sun throughout the day. They believe that the heat of rays of the sun would neutralise high temperature of the body that often may lead to precarious situations.[36]

A barren woman is considered so inauspicious that no other woman should take bath where she takes her bath. They blame the woman not the man in all cases. Fasting penances and other observances are aimed at the propitiation of several gods and goddess. Bathing in some holy river is done to remove barrenness.[37] Barrenness is regarded as a stigma and hence an unfortunate phenomenon. No scientific treatment is undertaken for its redemption. The only alternative for the issueless Kondh woman is to make a vow that she will offer a goat or a lamb for sacrifice during *Ghanta Parab* before the *Dharani Penu* in the event of birth of a child.[38]

Omens

Omens are used and interpreted to ascertain auspiciousness and inauspiciousness of certain objects whether animate or inanimate. Certain local birds-*kuguria*, *kumbhatal* and *gundru* are considered auspicious if seen on the way, while going to capture bird. The crowing of wild fowl (*joda kayu*) is auspicious as it brings more money for a man if he sells anything. Sight of a barren woman and fox crossing the path from left to right is viewed inauspicious.[39]

Totemism is a common feature of the Kondh population and they believe in their mysterious relation with some plants besides animals. Kondhs believe that the totemic plants and animals have helped or protected their respective ancestors of the clan or have proved to be of some peculiar use or service. They have shown reverence for totem objects and do not destroy them. They refrain from eating their fruits or flowers. A totemic object found in a condition of disease is nursed back to health and left free. The dead totemic plants and animals are given full honour and are attended to their last hour accordingly. In this connection Verrier Elwin has stated: "In India totemism has failed rather remarkably to exercise any influence on tribal art. Many tribals are still totemic in a faded sort of way and we might well have expected to find representation of the totem animal or plant on walls and pillars or at the very least in tattoo patterns. But this is not the case; you may go to a Gond house where the family totem is a dog or a Kondh house where it is a peacock".[40]

Religious functionaries in fact are the representatives of the people to propitiate god, deities and spirits with a full sense of reliance. They invoke these divine powers through ritual invocation, offering and sacrifices and thereby solicit blessings. The presence of the Kondh priest is required at the marriage ceremony, on the occasion of the naming of new born child, at funeral feasts and at all other domestic ceremonies. They have no special endowments in any form. They have only honourable places at all public and private festivals. They are paid by those who employ them or receive gifts from the community when religious ceremonies are conducted. Thus the Kondhs do not feel to attach much importance to priesthood. Gradually only one priest remains to worship their chief deity.[41]

In a Kondh village, the medicine man has his own importance like the priest, his office is not hereditary. The medicine man is prompted to begin his practice as a result of a series of spiritual experiences with a goddess who having guided him into his profession and remains thereafter his mentor and mediatress with the gods. He is respected by the tribe who regard him as one, specially chosen by a goddess. He is also accredited with possessing supernatural powers. The environment of the Kondhs plays a vital role for this. Due to ignorance, superstition and prejudice usually in case of sickness the *disari* or medicine man is summoned. He derives the cause of the disaster and prescribes the remedy which is mostly an animal sacrifice made with grain and liquor.

While on the one hand the Kondhs believe in supernatural causation of death and disaster, on the other hand they have an indigenous system of wealth which is primary based on use of wild herbs, obtained from forest. *Disari, jani, kutaka* and many other practitioners help them in curing several ailments.

A specialist is said to have theoretical, practical and above all divine wisdom. One cannot achieve his status, if any one of these qualities is lacked. Wisdom plays the most important role. Unless one is blessed with divine wisdom he cannot be a specialist. It is imparted to certain people in dreams and by communication with spiritual and supernatural beings. Religious headman is believed to be in possession of divine wisdom. Women have no access to general medical knowledge. They are only aware of certain medicines that are used specifically during birth, for contraception, abortion, amenorrhea and are also familiar with remedies for common ailments. Certain priests, shamans and sorcerers are believed to be able to communicate directly with gods and goddesses and acquire the divine wisdom.[42]

The Kondhs not only have deep faith in their god and goddess but also they fear the ghost of the dead called *duma*. Whenever anybody feels ill they believe that it is due to the curse of any spirit or violation of any taboo. They have their own doctors. They are still living in magic and by their magical performance they also cure many of their physical troubles. Before proper treatment they call upon the diviner to attend the patient for diagnosis. These religious functionaries worship the gods and goddess on behalf of the community in several occasions. They are the representatives of the people to propitiate gods, deities and spirits with a full sense of reliance. They invoke these divine powers through rituals, invocations, offerings and sacrifices and thereby solicit their blessings for the people. The religious functionaries invoke and invite the deities to action through incarnation. Invocations are sung in chorus by the *bejunis*. These are the praises for the supernatural powers.

Jani

Jani is the ritual head of the village. This post is hereditary. The office of the *jani* passes from the father to the eldest son. In case the *jani* has no son, his younger brother gets the chance. He performs all village rituals and is given a special share of sacrificial animal.

There are also village priestesses known as *janiyani*. Only a married woman is entitled to become *janiyani*. Once a woman becomes a *janiyani* she remains as such till her death. Even when she becomes a widow, she retains her powers. She too attends all the group rituals. It is believed that she goes into trance and at that moment she has possession of god or spirit. While she is in possession of godly power many of the villagers who have problems and difficulties approach her for reliefs.

Ichan Jani

The assistant of the *jani* is called *ichan jani* who sacrifices animals, arrange *puja* accessories if required, participate in the recitation of the incarnation along with the *jani*. This post is not hereditary but one of the male members of *jani's* lineage holds the post at the pleasure of the village council.

Pujari

The post of *pujari* is hereditary. In each village, there is a *pujari* who presides over *meriah/kedu* festival along with *jani*. He plays a different role. He prepares an umbrella out of bamboo collected from the forest in the dead night unnoticed by anybody. In the *meriah* procession he dangles the umbrella to ward off the evil eye of the pernicious spirits. He too chants spell with *jani*.[43]

Beju

Bejus or shamans are specialists in divination. In each village, there are two or three shamans. They are the specialists who derive their power from the supernatural agencies directly through mystic experience. They regularly worship and appease their own spirit. Through divination, prayer and rites, the *beju* gets into trance during which he visualises the reason causing harm to the people. During trance he talks with the spirit and requests them on behalf of the victim to free them from the troubles. When he regains sense, they adopt rice supplication process called *puchuna* through which shaman finds out the cause of the disease and specific vow to be made. *Puchana* is sometimes called for twice or more if the disease is not cured for a long period.[44]

The female shaman is called *bejuni*. They have their own adopted spirits to whom they regularly worship to get their favour and help in occult practices. They can communicate with spirits and deities who are believed to be responsible for causing human problems. Kondhs believe that shamanism is a magico-religious art which is gifted to certain persons by supernatural powers. Generally, the old women are eligible to become *bejuni*, though there is no formal age restriction. This is also not a hereditary profession. It is an acquired art and a personal accomplishment. Skill in dancing is essential for a *bejuni*. While doing so, she puts a red sari and uses metal bells at her ankles. She waves a bundle of peacock feather over the head of a sufferer to the accompaniment of dance and music. It is a preliminary step to appease the *Penu* (god) and in due course of frenzied dancing, she gets into a trance and in that state makes prophecies and offers solutions to the problems of the clients. Names of different *Penus* are also to be mugged up before becoming a *bejuni*. She also knows the art of divination with the movement of the winnowing-fan weaving of peacock feathers and supplication through *arua*-rice in the winnowing fan. Simultaneously, she knows the nature of sacrifice to be made for different diseases. To know all these techniques an apprentice undergoes training under a *bejuni*, called *pat bejuni* or head *bejuni*. Thus in a village there may be four to five *pat bejunis* who impart training to the interested candidates in the evening, after the day's work. The *bejunis* are believed to acquire power through the special grace of their own ancestor spirits or *penus*. It generally comes to the person who has a temperament towards it. With the increase of their earnestness or rather yearning and devotion, they begin to pass sleepless nights in contemplation of certain *Penus*. She has to observe certain steps of ceremony for this post. As a black magician her acts are secretly sought.[45]

Table 1 depicts various kinds of services rendered by the shamans and shamanin in different rituals.

Table 1: Classification of Shamanic Jobs Undertaken by the Bejus and Bejunis.

1. Diagnosis, curative and preventive practices for treatment of various kinds of illness.	(a) To determine cause and (b) To prescribe remedy for various kinds of fever, body aches and pains, small pox, chicken pox, unidentified diseases etc.	Individual family level
2. Dealing with deities and spirits (exorcism)	(a) To prevent and remove various types of diseases, misfortunes and human sufferings (other than diseases.) (b) To ward off malevolent spirits including (ancestral spirit) causing trouble. (c) To appease benevolent ones to earn their pleasure and protection. (d) To detect the spirit causing trouble.	Individual family level
3. Performance of life cycle rituals	(a) Pregnancy and child birth- To prevent miscarriage infant death, and facilitate easy delivery. To identify the ancestor taking rebirth in the new born baby. (b) Puberty rites for girls to ward off evil spirits. (c) Preventive rites during wedding to protect the couple from malevolent spirits. (d) To detect the cause and agencies responsible for abnormal and unnatural deaths and prescribe ritual remedies to prevent future mishaps.	Individual family level

Source: A.K. Gomango and S.C. Mohanty, "Festivals, Rituals and Shamans among the Dongria Kandha", *Adivasi*, Vol. 48, No. 2, December 2008, SCSTRTI, Bhubaneswar, 16.

The service of the *bejuni* is required more in case of sterility and miscarriage. They also attend problems of child delivery and post delivery periods. She participates actively in the ritual after the birth of the new born. She sacrifices fowl and pigeon in this ceremony.

The onset of first menstruation of a girl is treated as a period of crisis in the Kondh society. In this period, the girl is considered vulnerable and susceptible to the attack of malevolent deities, spirits and evil eye. Therefore she is subjected to certain taboos and restrictions as a preventive measure. The *beju* is called to perform certain rituals to appease the deity called *Gangu Penu* who can help for the betterment of the family and ward off the evil eye. In normal cases of death, the *bejuni* have no role to play.[46] But in unusual and unnatural deaths caused by suicide, snake-bite, small-pox, cholera, pregnancy, delivery and tiger attack the role of the *bejuni* is quite important. She has to conduct protective and preventive rituals for identifying and appeasing the concerned supernatural agencies. In the Kondh society, beliefs and practices connected with religion and shamanism go side by side. It cannot be separated. Shamanism is strongly linked with their socio-economic and religious life.

Disari

Disari is always a man, since women are not entitled to hold this status. The *disari* uses his divine wisdom for spiritual healing purposes and he is familiar with the use of herbal medicine for various ailments. *Disari* knows the transformation of souls, and therefore, is regarded as the bearer of knowledge in his society. He gets medical knowledge, the method of diagnosis and procedure for worship and sacrifice to be held for healing purpose from the deity in his dream.

He is a medicine man. He applies herbal medicines which are charged with magical powers. His post is not hereditary. The *Dongrias* believe the position of the *disari* is granted by the gods and goddesses along with divine wisdom. The chief function of the *disari* is to determine auspicious moments via astrological prediction. For example, the day of worship for festivals such as *meriah*, *ghanta parva* and *mandiarani*. His knowledge of medicine is also considered to be god given wisdom. When attempting to cure a patient, he uses a combination of religious chanting, herbal medicine and occasionally religious rituals with sacrifices. The *disari* knows about the transformation of souls.

Sisa

The assistant to the *disari* is known as *sisa*. He follows the commands of the *disari* on all occasions and is also taught only by him. More than one *sisa* works under a *disari*. As a rule the *sisa* can assist *disari* but he may take over his charge after his death. He also seeks divine wisdom himself when the gods and goddess are satisfied with him. They endow him with divine or spiritual wisdom. From *disari, sisa* learns about the medicinal plants and their use. He also learns about the application of various medicines and diagnoses diseases. His knowledge includes the characteristics of gods and goddesses and astrology.[47]

Kutaka

Kutia Kondh considers that anything harmful to man's health and fortune is due to the activities of certain evil spirits. They are the traditional believers on the efficacy of magico-religious rites. This act is generally performed by the sorcerers. The sorcerer of the Kutia Kondh society is called *kutaka*. When a Kutia suffers from any sorts of illness, he first consults with *kutaka*. The *kutaka* first of all finds all the causes and the spirit responsible for the disease. Then he starts treatment by all means of some magical rites followed by sacrifice of a bird or animal as per the gravity of the disease and the spirit.[48]

Religion plays an important role in the social life of Kondhs. The social laws, customs and rites of their society are well connected with their religion. In Kondh society, violation of oath is believed to be invariably punished by divine wrath. They believe that first duty which god has imposed upon them is hospitality. Persons guilty of the neglect of established observances are punished by divine wrath, either during their current lives or in the next birth. The penalties are death, poverty, disease, loss of children and other forms of calamities. Kondhs worship all deities of their own tribe, *Bura Penu* to the orthodox Hindu Goddess *Kali* and *Durga*. Generally the Kondhs worship no images and they have no temples. The stream, the rock, the grove, the glen and the sky above them constitute the Kondh shrine.[49] The animals such as buffalo, cow, goat, lamb, pig, fowl and pigeon are mainly sacrificed. Egg is also a sacrificial item. All the rituals are directed towards stimulating natural process. Illness and misfortune is attributed to displeasure of the god, goddess and also ancestors. The sacrifice of different kinds of animals and birds is considered appropriate appeasement. Religion and magic are the two ways of hiding over crisis. The magic and religion are very close to each other. Actually, there is no magician in Kondh society. Only the *bejunis* who are the specialists, perform some techniques to appease their respective guardian spirit by performing appropriate rituals and sacrifices. On the festive occasions, the Kondhs worship the dead ancestors (*duma*) who are represented by wooden posts in the house known as *tuli munda*. Besides this, the Kondhs worship many deities at different periods of time. Their festivals are linked with agriculture and health problems. They believe in efficacy of magic. Good fortune is ascribed to white or good magic and black or bad magic is ascribed to misfortune. Unnatural events, accidents and infections are related to black magic. So they conduct many festivals for the betterment of their life.

Their belief on ancestral spirit forces them to accept that ancestors appear in dream when they desire to receive periodic worship. They are fatalists and believe in chance and luck.[50]

In fact, the beliefs of Kondh are dominated by animistic and fatalistic orientations. Their supernatural rites are explicitly directed towards happiness and security in the world and to ward off danger as well as evil. They believe that untoward events occur in life due to wrath of god. Gods and goddesses, presiding deities and spirits are only approachable through special functions.

Kondhs neither worship image nor build temples. The symbols of the deities are rough stones and logs placed under a lofty *sal* or *mohuli* tree. Religion forms the hard core of Kondh culture and associated with every aspect of their day to day life and socio-cultural practices. They follow certain principles and festivals to worship their gods and goddesses for the cure and prevention of diseases.

Ghanta Parba

This festival is observed commonly in the month of *Baisakh* for three days. In this festival *Hira Penu, Takrani Penu* and *Kudi Penu* are worshipped. *Jani* and *pat-bejuni* worship the god and goddess in this function. As *pat-bejuni* has to keep an earthen pot *(ghanta)* over her head, this festival is called *Ghanta Parva*. This ritual continues for three days. It is believed that after this ritual people may not suffer from small pox and cholera in future.[51]

Korubiha Dakina

It is otherwise known as *meriah puja*. It is the biggest festival observed at community level. It is observed once in every five years. In this festival *Kutia Kondhs* were sacrificing human beings in the past but now it is substituted by goat/cock. The sacrificed animal is offered to *Dharani Penu* with the belief to ensure better crop, immunity from the diseases. They also believe that by observing this festival the community may be saved from unforeseen calamities.

Badabiha Dakina

This festival is observed to cure a serious disease of a person. It is observed on a Monday in the month of *Chaitra* (March-April). This festival is observed by the individual household of the village who has taken a vow to appease the goddess, *Kamati Penu* to cure the serious illness of a member of the family. The *kutaka* of the village performs the rituals in front of the house of the vow-taker. A goat or a sheep is sacrificed to appease the deity during this ritual. The flesh of the sacrificed animal is distributed among the households of the village.[52]

Badbinere

Badbinere is celebrated annually in *Dasehara Lanju* and *Chaita Lanju*. In this, two malevolent deities *Kamati Penu* and *Mardi Penu* are invoked, worshipped and bidden farewell. This festival is intended to encourage the departure of malevolent deities. These deities create some problems for human beings. If not properly satisfied, they cause spots or wounds by small pox, chicken pox and measles.

Dasehra Kandanga Dakine

It is celebrated in the month of September/October. *Takurani Penu* and *Kamati Penu* are offered a *puja* in the village. It ensures people's social wellbeing and mitigates epidemic.[53]

Dakandi Palukandi

This is an invocation to the gods, a common method of treatment involving intervention of the gods or divine healing. It is generally used for children and also for adults, particularly as a cure for women disease. It is an effective treatment for the exorcism of evil spirits from body and mind, snake-bite, fever and injuries.

The practitioner first chants in his language and invokes deities from all corners. A small chicken is required to be sacrificed. He defines the cause as either the patient has ignored the deities or because the patient has neglected to pray them. So the *kutaka* now tries his level best to satisfy the deities.

The preparations for *ash dakina* are made well in advance and persons having sufficient knowledge of medicinal plants are assigned to collect herbs and plants under the direction of the main priests to prepare medicine.

Eju Penu Dakina

It is another ritual performed to cure diseases caused by evil spirits. If a husband or a wife is sick for a long time then his partner arranges an act of worship and presents an offering to the water god in return for the life of the patient. This ritual is organised on Sunday at a place where water can be found. It is believed that water god washes away the patient's sufferings. The thorns of the *bela mara* or *bela* tree (Aegle marmelos), *tuturi mara* or *ankranti* (Solanum Xenthocarpum) and *tade mara* or ripe banana (Musa sapientum) plants are the usual requirements for the ritual.

Wechinja

Wechinja is a method of treatment that includes various rites described below. The *kutaka* only applies his supernatural power. It is commonly used to cure aches and pains affecting the head, stomach and chest. He first identifies the painful area and then places his thumb on it while chanting. He then puts an arrow. *Kutak* chews on the shafts of the arrow until he draws out blood and insects. By identifying the insect, he can establish the nature of illness and the identity of the god responsible for causing pain. If a patient suffers from headache, an insect resembling the honeybee is extracted, while the appearance of a long tail insect signifies stomach troubles. The extraction of honeybee proves that *Mara Penu* is responsible for the pain.

Jaka Dakandi (Top Worship)

In *Jaka Dakandi* there are two sites of offering to *Yama Penu* (the demon god) one, outside the patient's house and the other, inside the house where the patient is sleeping. Only a thread is extended from the arrow (placed outside) through the roof, down to the patient. On the end of the thread that is dropped down to the patient, a leaf from a *pipada mara* or *Jari* (Ficus scandens) is tied. This leaf must remain suspended over the head of the patient but should not touch him/ her inside the house. The healer chants near the patient.

If the *Yam Penu* feels happy with the invocation and prayer then he asks for a sacrifice. To give the patient life, another life has to be sacrificed. At that point *Yam Penu* requests the *Linga Penu* (god of creation) to "give life to" or cure the patient. The *Linga Penu* then gives life to the patient by passing it through the thread which is extended down to the leaf to the patient's body.

When the patient is more serious and difficult to save life then the ritual is performed on the roof of the patient's house. The magic healer sacrifices a black hen and follows a difficult method to appease *Yam Penu*. A fistful of earth is placed on a bamboo mat made of 14 interwoven bamboo strips. A line of turmeric powder is then drawn and some rice grains are placed at its centre. The four edges of mat are smeared with ash from the hearth and an arrow is placed vertically above the ash. On one end a branch of *pipada mara* or *Jari* (ficus scandens) is tied. It is believed that this will satisfy *Yam Penu*, as he will then order the *Linga Penu* (birth god) to restore life (*jella*) by means of the leaves of ficus scandens.[54]

Asa Dakina

Lada Penu is the first deity to be invoked when an epidemic breaks out or the health of the entire community is threatened specially during monsoon when gastro intestinal disorders and diarrhoea are common. In such cases, traditional ritual known as *Asa Dakina* or medicinal plant worship is carried out in the hope of preserving the community's health.[55]

Lodang

Lodang is a *puja* offered to the specific deity after a person is cured from a disease. The vowed sacrifice is offered for the cured person. *Arua* rice, *Bel* leaves, *Mandara* leaves, vermilion, winnowing fan, fire pot, oil and promised sacrificial animal are required for *Lodang*. In most of the cases the sacrificial animal is a hen. The cured person sits near the *beju* throughout the *puja*. He holds the animal and makes it eat a few grains of the ritual rice from his palm. The *puja* takes two or three hours time on the following morning, the sacrificial animal is taken to the hill stream. After some rituals, the animal is killed and the blood is offered to the specific god or deity.[56]

Other invocations

Women suffering from water retention like dropsy are instructed to worship *Gangi Penu* at a site where water is found. The worship involves the sacrifice of a piglet and a twig of *Pipada*

(Ficus scandens) placed at the worship sight believed to drive away evil spirits. The prescribed medicine is the root of *Patala garuda* plant (Rauvolfia serpentina).

The worship of *Gangi Penu* is necessary in the treatment of leprosy. Leprosy is regarded as a form of punishment by a village god *(Deukuda)*. The bark of *raga mara* (a species visible only to the *Kutaka* at the time of need) is prescribed. Sometimes the healer shows his unwillingness to cure the patient by pretending that *raga mara* is unavailable.[57] When the first conception is realised in the third month, the priest of the daughter-in-law's village is invited to the son-in-law's village for the ritual to sacrifice a goat (*boda*). The message is usually sent by the husband or by any of the in-law's family. The offering known as *Siruki Bakada*, is observed. It can be held on any day except Thursday and Saturday. The belief is that if the family deities are not propitiated they may bring harm to the unborn child.[58] Likewise a barren woman performs many rituals and offers sacrifices while longing for a child.

Kondhs believe that more diseases are caused by evil spirits, which enter the body through the medium of air, water or plants. The witch doctors have the capacity to identify, influence and control those powerful forces. Kondh's concept of diseases and their cure is therefore based on an interaction of man and sprit. Supernatural beings play a benevolent role in their daily lives. Human suffering is attributed to the malevolent powers of the supernatural. It is believed that supernatural powers dominate human beings but a witch doctor's skill is able to counteract or defeat these malevolent powers. This forms the hard core of Kondh culture. The socio-cultural dimension of health in one sense is a myth, in other context it is a reality. Thus if a tribal group worships to get cure from disease, it is assumed that they are all superstitious but perhaps it is forgotten that same thing is performed also in the so-called modern society. The question of rationality cannot be judged or examined in isolation, without examining the ecosystem, health facilities available and socio-economic conditions. However socio-cultural tradition plays an important role in the context of health and treatment.[59]

Kondhs are poly-theists and worship gods, goddesses, deities, spirits and other natural objects. Each of these is intimately connected with different aspects of life. However, their beliefs and practices are dearer to them. The various divinities in the Kondh pantheon form the basis of the tribal philosophy and ideals. There is a strong conviction that all worldly needs can only be satisfied by the mercy of unseen powers. Indeed the common beliefs, customs, traditions, values and practices of Kondhs are intimately connected with their concept of health, disease and its cure.

References

1. Jose Boban K. *Tribal Ethnomedicine: Continuity and Change*, A.P.H. Publishing Corporation, New Delhi, 1998, 268.
2. *Ibid.,* 133-134.
3. S.P. Gupta, "Tribal Concept of Health, Disease and Remedy", in Buddhadeb Chaudhuri (ed.), *Tribal Health Socio-Cultural Dimension*, Inter-India Publication, New Delhi, 1986, 161.
4. Jose Boban K., *op. cit.*, 12.
5. *The Kandha of Orissa*, Scheduled Castes and Scheduled Tribes Research and Training Institute, (herein after SCSTRTI), Bhubaneswar, 2006, 179-183.
6. Mihir Kumar Jena, Padmini Pathi, Kamala Kumari Patnaik and Klaus Seeland, *Forest Tribes of Orissa*, Vol. 2, *Kuttia Kondh*, D.K. Print World, New Delhi, 2006, 150.
7. *The Kandha of Orissa*, SCSTRTI, *op. cit.*, 268-269.
8. N.R. Patnaik, *History and Culture of Khond Tribe*, Commonwealth Publisher, New Delhi, 1992, 203.
9. *Ibid.,* 210.
10. Mihir Kumar Jena, Padmini Pathi, Jagganath Dash, Kamala Kumari Patnaik and Klaus Seeland, *Forest Tribes of Orissa*, Vol. 1, *Dongaria Kondh*, D.K. Print World, New Delhi, 2002, 191-192.
11. *Ibid.*, 196-197.
12. Mihir Kumar Jena, *et al.*, *Kuttia Kondh*, *op. cit.*, 113.
13. Mihir Kumar Jena, *et al.*, *Dongaria Kondh*, *op. cit.*, 217.
14. Mihir Kumar Jena, *et al.*, *Kuttia Kondh*, *op. cit.*, 114.
15. *Ibid.,* 139.
16.. *Ibid.*, 256-259.
17. *The Kandha of Orissa,* SCSTRTI, *op. cit.,* 207-208.
18. Mihir Kumar Jena, *et al.*, *Kuttia Kondh, op. cit.*, 203-204.
19. Mihir Kumar Jena, *et al.*, *Dongaria Kondh, op. cit.*, 128-130.
20. *Ibid.,* 55-57.
21. *The Kandha of Orissa,* SCSTRTI, *op. cit.,* 206.

22. *Ibid.*, 154.
23. P.K. Mohanty, *Encyclopedia of Schedule Tribes in India*, Vol. 4, East, Isha Books, Delhi, 2006, 174.
24. *The Kandha of Orissa,* SCSTRTI, *op. cit*, 257-259.
25. Mihir Kumar Jena, *et al., Dongaria Kondh, op. cit.,* 67.
26. G. Bulliyya, "Indigenous Health Care Practices among the Kondh"- in Awadesh N. Sharma, *et al.,* (ed.), *Indigenous Health Care and Ethno Medicine*, Sarup and Sons, New Delhi, 2006, 60.
27. *The Kandha of Orissa*, SCSTRTI, *op. cit.,* 148-149.
28. Saraswati Swain, "Tradition and Customs Associated with Pregnancy and Child Birth among Kondhs of Phulbani." *Adivasi* Vol. XXIX No. 324, September and December, 1989, Tribal and Harijan Research and Training Institute (herein after THRTI), Bhubaneswar, 16-17.
29. *The Kandha of Orissa,* SCSTRTI, *op. cit.,* 27.
30. N.R. Patnaik, *op. cit.,* 168.
31. *Ibid.,* 170-172.
32. Mihir Kumar Jena, *et al., Dongria Kondh, op. cit.,* 55.
33. Almas Ali, "Health Status of the Tribals in India: An Overview", in Dipak Kumar Adak, *et al.*, (eds.), *Demography and Health Profile of the Tribals*, Anmol Publication, New Delhi, 2003, 10.
34. N.K. Behura and K.K. Mohanty, *Tribal Orissa, Reading in Social Anthropology*, Dominant Publisher, New Delhi, 2006, 118.
35. N.R. Patnaik, *op. cit*, 166-167.
36. G. Bulliyya, *op. cit.*, 61.
37. P.K. Mohanty, *op. cit.*, 17.
38. *The Kandha of Orissa*, SCSTRTI, *op. cit.*, 147.
39. *Ibid.,* 207.
40. Verrier Elwin, *The Tribal Art of Middle India*, London, 1951, 110.
41. W.W. Hunter, *A Statistic Account of Bengal,* Vol. XIX, London, 1877, 94-95.
42. Mihir Kumar Jena, *et al., Dongaria Kondh, op. cit.,* 122-123.
43. *The Kandha of Orissa,* SCSTRTI, *op. cit.*, 187-188.

44. N. Patnaik, F. Bara and A. Mall, "Herbal Medicines of Dongrias" *Adivasi,* Vol. XXVI, No. 4, December, 1986, SCSTRTI, Bhubaneswar, 1.
45. Prabhansu Sekhar Das Pattnaik, "Bejuni, Their Initiation into Shamanhod", *Adivasi,* Vol. XIV, No. 1, THRTI, Bhubaneswar, 1972-73, 12.
46. A.K. Gomango and S.C. Mohanty, "Festival Rituals and Shamans Among the Dongria Kondh", *Adivasi* Vol. 48, No. 2, December, 2008, SCSTRTI, Bhubaneswar, 16.
47. Mihir Kumar Jena, *et al., Dongria kondh, op. cit.,* 125-126.
48. *The Kandha of Orissa,* SCSTRTI, *op. cit.,* 287.
49. N.R. Patnaik, *op.cit.*, 222-225.
50. P.S. Daspatnaik, "Kandha", *Tribes of Orissa*, SCSTRTI, Bhubaneswar, Orissa Government Press, 2004, 164.
51. *The Kandha of Orissa,* SCSTRTI, *op. cit.*, 192-193.
52. *Ibid.*, 271-273.
53. Mihir Kumar Jena, *et al., Kuttia Kondh, op. cit.*, 146-149.
54. *Ibid.,* 262-265.
55. Mihir Kumar Jena, *et al., Dongaria Kondh, op. cit.,* 187.
56. N. Pattnaik, *(et.al.), op. cit.*, 1.
57. Mihir Kumar Jena, *et al., Kuttia Kondh, op. cit.*, 265-266.
58. Manoranjan Acharya, "Rituals Associated with Child Birth Among Kondhs", *Adavasi*, XXVI, No. 2, April-June, 1986, SCSTRTI, Bhubaneswar, 15.
59. Buddhadeb Chaudhuri, *Health, Forest and Development*: *The Tribal Situation*, Inter-India Publication, New Delhi, 2003, 39.

4

Diseases and Medicines

Man is a unique creation of God. Like other living beings, man has been provided with food, water and shelter around his habitat. Human beings are different from other living organisms since they have the capacity to reason and this basic reasoning ability made human beings to devise ways for the best use of land, their plants and plant extracts to its fullest benefit. The relationship between man and plants is an age old phenomenon. Man has been using plants for various purposes such as food, fodder, clothing, shelter etc. from pre-historic times. Above all, plants are friendly and beautiful. They are the largest and longest living immobile organisms and often an amazing diversity of forms. Primitive human beings stepped out of the Stone Age carnivorism and started using plants found around their settlement. Medicinal values of various plants were primarily assessed by them through hit and trial method. Plants are integral parts of nature. Nature reflects in them the creative power of god. The physical beauty and its chemistry are of immense importance to humankind. They are life sustaining force on earth. Herbal drugs obtained from plants are believed to be much safer, fresh and proves elixir in the treatment of various ailments.[1]

The history of use of plants and animals as a source of medicine dates back perhaps to the origin of human race. In the pre-historic era, early man lived in the forests in the constant fear of natural calamities and dreaded diseases. The identification of useful plants and animals available in nature had commenced in the pre-historic times. Out of his inherent instincts, man tried to develop certain techniques to survive from natural disasters and used various plant parts, animal organs and few minerals to cure the diseases he suffered from. Miraculously in some cases, he succeeded in getting good results and developed an indigenous system of treatment.[2]

In India, reference to plants is found in the *Rig-Veda* and it is the earliest record of plants for use as medicine. It has an encyclopedia of tried, tested, trusted history of medicinal plants and traditional medical practices. The medicines mentioned in the *Charaka Samhita* and the *Susruta Samhita* is esteemed as treasures of literature on indigenous medicines. Even today, the system of allopathy is still unknown to the tribals inhabiting in the interior areas. Most of the tribals of rural and urban areas depend on ayurvedic or traditional folk medicines to cure various diseases. The traditional medicines provide health service to 70 to 80 per cent of world population. In recent times emphasis has been given to collect information on ethno-medicinal uses of plants from various parts of the world. It is estimated that 2000 drugs have been used to cure human ailments in India. Out of these around 200 are of animal origin and another 200 are of mineral origin and the rest are of plant origin. Tribal people are the real powerhouse of traditional herbal knowledge. These indigenous people have been involved in doing herbal practices since time immemorial for curing various health disorders. They are the real custodian of medicinal plants. All this traditional knowledge of medicine was present only in oral form and are transmitted from generation to generation. Some medicinal herbs are believed to cure practically every human disease from head to toe. The tribals' concept of disease, health, medicine, traditional health institutions, practices and overall health behaviours are in fact manifestations of their cultural response to this dimension of their material and non-material existence.[3]

Health, hygiene, sickness, diagnosis and disease treatment comprise a vital sector of human society. But tribals including Kondhs consider disease as pernicious and detrimental to normal life. It is certainly a departure from the normal state of health.

Tribals do not consider any disease as the cause of neglect of body or its organs. They consider disease as an integral part of life process. They believe that diseases cause both transient and intransient illness, and disease means unhappiness, fear, tragedy, expenditure, suffering and ultimately death.[4]

The common customs, traditions, values, beliefs and practices associated with the tribe's health and diseases have a direct bearing on their treatment of physical ailments, besides other socio-psychological reasons. From a traditional medicine man or witchdoctor a tribal patient does not merely receive a physical health treatment but something much more than that. He gets socio-psychological reinforcements which he cannot get from modern medical practitioners. These reinforcements are based on the understanding of traditional beliefs and practices of the community. The tribal medicine has its own etiological aspects which may be classified into two broad areas, such as supernatural and physical. The supernatural aspect forms a part of belief system of the people and they accordingly take resort to magico-religious practices of healing. In tribal societies, the etiology includes breach of taboo, supernatural vengeance of gods, ghosts and evil spirits, ghost/spirit intrusion, evil eye, witchcraft, sorcery etc. The causes for some diseases are also attributed to physical factors such as hazards of weather, wrongful intake of food and beverages, etc. The disease causation and healing practices differ from one society to other because of human diversity and variation of socio-cultural factors. It is not desirable to question the belief system of the people but to examine the rational, irrational, non-rational aspects of human behaviour pertaining to health and ill health.

The principal ingredients of tribal medicine are derived from plant source. Various types of plants and herbs available in nature are collected for medicinal purposes, rather than, culturing or domesticating them. Such medicinal plants and herbs are identified and collected by medicine man. He is the only person who is supposed to collect the medicinal plants and prepare medicine out of them. He is specially equipped with the knowledge of diseases and medicines required. The medicines are not preserved as they believe that fresh collected plants are more effective than dried ones. The medicine man maintains the secrecy involved in medicinal preparations. Various parts of plants and herbs such as branches, fruits, buds, flowers, leaves, barks, roots and offshoots have specific use for treatment of diseases. There are prescriptions, prohibitions and taboos for collection of plants and herbs on specific day and time. It is also believed if a particular plant or herb or part thereof is not collected on prescribed date and time, it looses its medicinal value. Some plants and herbs are stored and preserved for future use whereas some others require fresh applications. The plants and herbs are often semi-processed for medicinal use. The medicinemen are conversant with the preparation of a single or a multiple number of plants and herbs for preparation of medicines. As per the disease some such medicines are administered orally, or applied externally. Some parts of plants and herbs are kept outside or inside the house for their repellent effect to prevent certain diseases. Besides plants and herbs, the tribal medicinemen also utilise objects of animal origin and mineral origin to treat various types of diseases.[5]

The Kondhs in general, along with other tribes, opine that the causes of sickness are either supernatural or physical. They agree fully with other tribes that the supernatural causative agents are (i) breach of taboo, (ii) sorcery, (iii) spirit intrusion, (iv) evil eye, (v) wrath of gods and goddesses and (vi) ghost intrusion; whereas the physical causative agents are (i) effect of weather, (ii) effect of wrong food, (iii) contact with certain living organisms, (iv) blood getting impure, (v) accidents and natural calamities and (vi) unknown causes. The tribal people have pharmacopoeia of their own for their manifold diseases, like malaria, yaws, leprosy, scabies, venereal disease, bowel complains influenza, cholera, small pox, etc.[6]

Kondhs of Odisha depend upon forestry and simple agriculture. The commodities used by them for every day use is mostly forest produce and agricultural corps. They also depend upon forest for their medicines. As the children of forest, they consider the forest as their home. During our fieldwork we got interesting observations regarding this. When we asked "what forest is for you?" The reply was "*Jada ma bagatiki bale*", which means forest is everything for us.[7] It proves how so far they depend upon forest for their life. Due to their constant association with the forest for meeting their everyday requirements, Kondhs have developed an intimate knowledge of the use of wild plants in various aspects of their life. Their medicinemen have real knowledge about the value of plants.

Tribal medicinemen are individuals of excellence known by different names in different tribal societies. They play a vital role in catering to the healthcare needs of millions of tribal population. Their own community recognises them as competent to provide healthcare by using bio-resources and mineral substance. They use some methods that have a support from religious beliefs to cure people suffering from various diseases and disabilities. They are the carriers of healing traditions, which have been orally transmitted from generation to generation. They are the knowledgeable persons who directly use the medicinal herbs, roots and other parts of the plants for healing treatment. These carriers of tribal health traditions have survived over thousands of years in spite of a total lack of documentation and any institutional framework to support and sustain them.[8]

The Kondhs believe that diseases are caused by evil spirits. They become angry and do harm if one has not propitiated them properly. Thus to a Kondh the real enemies of human health and prosperity are the gods and the evil spirits. The usual theory of disease in the Kondh society is that it is caused by the breach of some taboo or by the anger of hostile spirits and ghosts of the dead. Sickness is the routine punishment for every lapse and crime done by them. Accordingly, they have taboos and prayers. Invoking the blessings of gods and propitiating the evil spirits are necessary to have a smooth and healthy life. The *Jani* or the village priest in addition to his religious functions acts as mediator between the people and the mystical power. He prays and offers alcoholic drink and blood of sacrificial animals. By these he tries to maintain a good relationship between the people on the one hand and the mystical power on the other hand. Thus Kondhs resort to magico-religious treatment of diseases caused by supernatural and human agencies.

Besides, the supernatural causes, the Kondhs also believe in natural causes of some common diseases like fever, cold, cough, headache, stomach pain, toothache, cut, burn, snake and insect bite etc. Yet their emphasis on the supernatural power puts low threshold on the awareness of disease and pain, encouraging them to tolerate and accept. They do not care much for the common diseases unless it becomes very severe and inflict acute pain to the affected person. People very often use more than one plant as medicine for a particular disease. Sometimes a plant is used for more than one disease[9]

Most of the traditional medicines are prepared from the fresh plant material collected from the wild. However, some of the plant materials (annuals, fruits, flowers etc.) are collected during the periods of availability. These materials are sun dried or stored for use as and when necessary. The dried plant materials are used for the preparation of medicine generally in the form of powder. The fresh materials are used in the form of paste, or the juice is extracted and used. Animal organs are also added for good results wherever required. Animal organs such as teeth, bones, etc. are collected and stored at the time of availability and used at the time of necessity. Plant parts are crushed manually using a cylindrical stone roller-pin locally called *Pua* and a flat rectangular stone base called *Sila*.[10]

The following are the diseases commonly found with the tribal people specifically the Kondhs. Use of specific plants for medicine, mode of preparation of drugs and its administration are provided below along with the disease.

Fever

Fever is the most common disease from which the Kondhs suffer frequently. They believe in two types of fever namely *Nomberi* and *Dadi* or *Pali nomberi*. The leaves of *Sapta* (Manilkara zapota), *Bhuinimbo* (Andrographis paniculata) plant and root of *Pitakeruan* (Holarrhena pubescens) are pounded together to extract juice. This juice is heated to make lukewarm. About half a cup of this juice is orally administered daily in an empty stomach early in the morning till the fever is cured.[11] Likewise, the root powder of *Bichuati* (Laportea interrupta) with *Golamaricha* (Piper nigrum) is orally administered with water to cure intermittent fever. Root is tied on right hand with a thread to cure cold fever and intermittent fever. Pallets made from the plant leaf of *Gayasa* (Leucas aspera) and *Golamaricha* (Piper nigrum) is also prescribed for seven days in empty stomach to cure cold fever. Besides a piece of root of *Chitakutei* (Euphorbia hirta) dipped in turmeric paste is tied on left hand to get relief from intermittent fever and cold fever. Decoction of root of *Pippali* (Piper longum), rhizome of lotus and stem of *Rakta Chandan* (Pterocarpus santalinus) is taken with one cup of cow urine in empty stomach for seven days during intermittent fever and fever due to cold.[12] Decoction of bark of *Koniyari* (Cascabela thevetia) is an effective medicine to reduce fever. Decoction of leaves of *Kanda koli* (Carissa carandas) is consumed to remit high fever.[13]

Nail infection

Latex of *Koniyari* (Cascabela thevetia) is applied to cure nail infection.[14]

Besides, they apply flower paste of *Dalimba* (Punica granatum) roasted with mustard oil to get cured from nail infection.[15]

Cold

The Kondh term for cold is *losom*. It is recognised by the symptoms of heavy flow of watery cough like substance from nose, giddiness and feeling of restlessness and cold sensation accompanied by aching of the limbs.

In continued and severe cases of cold, Kondhs use the paste of the root of *Ketkaya* (Pandanus fascicularis). They dilute the paste in water and 2 to 3 spoons of this diluted water is orally administered twice a day till cure. In addition to, the bark of *Sajana* (Moringa oleifera) tree is grated and boiled with water. The steam of this boiling water is inhaled for some time and then the cooled water is filtered to be orally administered.[16] Leaf juice of *Basanga* (Justicia adhatoda) long pepper powder and two tea spoon honey is also taken in empty stomach for 2 to 3 days to cure cough and cold.[17] Besides this, flowers and juice of fresh bark of *Kumbhi* (Careya arborea) is also taken with honey to cure cold.[18] In case of severe cold, bark of *Sajana* (Moringa oleifera) pounded with *Tulsi* (Ocimum sanctum) and *Sunthi* (Zangibar officinale) is taken twice a day. In the same case, they take the paste of *Peepalli* (Piper longum), *Ada* (Zangibar officinale) and *Tulsi* (Ocimum sanctum) along with honey twice a day.[19]

Cough

The Kondh term for cough is *Tanha*. It is recognised by cough, cold and irritation in the throat. Whenever it continues for longer period and becomes acute, they use different kinds of herbal medicines.

It can be noted here, the juice of *Mania* (Curculigo orchioides) and *Ada* (Zingiber officinale) is pounded together and the juice is squeezed on a small dish. About 2/3 spoonful of this juice is orally administered daily once for 3 to 4 days. In some cases, half burnt Ada (Zingiber officinale) is chewed by them. Mixed juice from leaf of *Tulsi* (Ocimum sanctum), *Ada* (Zingiber officinale) and honey also administrated as a medicine for cough. *Harida* (Terminalia chebula) fruit is boiled and made lukewarm and then about half a cup of this water is orally administered to the patient suffering from cough.[20]

The root of *Gai-gobaria* (Costus speciosus) is also given to cure cough. Water mixed with dry powder of the fruit of *Bahada*

(Terminalia bellirica) is taken to cure cough, cold and throat infection.[21] Decoction of the fruit *Harida* (Terminalia Chebula) is also taken to cure cough. Root powder of *Puruni* (Boerhavia diffusa) with equal amount of sugar candy is also taken to cure cough. Plant decoction of *Ankranti* (Solanum xanthocarpum) and *Pippali* (Piper longum) root powder are taken daily in empty stomach to cure cold, cough and fever.[22] The decoction of *Satabari* (Asparagus racemosus) is taken 3 to 4 times daily to cure cough and cold. Flower of *Arakh* (Calotropis gigantea) fried with a little ghee is taken to reduce cold, cough and asthma. This is taken once in a day till cure. Flower and juice of fresh bark of *Kumbhi* (Careya arborea) is taken with honey to soften the cough as an expectorant. Roots of *Akanbindi* (Cissampelos pareira) are pounded and taken to get relief from cough and cold. This is normally taken thrice daily.[23]

Entire plant of *Ankranti* (Solanum xanthocarpum) is boiled with bark of *Basang* (Justicia adhatoda) in half liter of water. The concentrated juice is filtered and the filtrate mixed with powder of *Pippli* (Piper longum) is given to cure cough.[24] Oil extracted from the nut of *Kalabhaliya* (Semecarpus anacardium) is applied on the pharyngeal wall with the help of a long stick in alternate day for cough and pharyngitis. Decoction of fruit of *Ankranti* (Solanum xanthocarpum) is also taken orally to cure cough. In case of severity, the fruits are taken orally by chewing.[25]

Tuberculosis

Decoction of fruits of *Ankranti* (Solanum xanthocarpum) is an effective indigenous medicine for tuberculosis.[26] The powered mixture of *Haladi* (Curcuma longa), *Bahada* (Terminalia bellirica) and *Harida* (Terminalia chebula) is also taken by the patient twice daily. Mixture of *Asoka* (Saraca asoca) bark, *Aparajeeta* (Cliteria ternatea) and *Jaitri* (Myristica fragrans) is prescribed for such patients to be taken thrice daily.[27] The patient suffering from tuberculosis is given leaf paste of *Basanga* (Justicia adhatoda) with *Golamaricha* (Piper nigrum) and he/she is advised to sleep in the goat shed. They prepare a *Pachana* with different parts of plants viz. bark of *Pitakeruan* (Holarrhena pubescens), root of *Utuli* (Pergularia daemia), root of *Kuilekha* (Hygrophila auriculata), leaf of *Apamaranga* (Achyranthes aspera), *Akanabindi* (Cissampelos pareira), root of *Dankari* (Mallotus repandus), *Guluchi* leaves (Tinospora cordifolia), *Harida* (Terminalia chebula), *Bahada* (Terminalia bellirica) alongwith *Amla* (Phyllanthus emblica) and

Peepalli (Piper longum) and this is given twice daily to the patient till cure.[28]

Skin Disease

In the decoction made from 50 gm. seed of the plant *Apamaranga* (Achyranthes aspera) with 10 gm. fresh *Bhrungaraj* (Eclipta prostrata) leaves in one liter water, 250 ml. of sesame oil is added and boiled to reduce it to 250 ml., which is applied to stop hair fall, lies and dandruff. This oil also cures scabies, itches, eczema and different types of skin diseases. One cup leaf extract of this plant mixed with 10 gm. of refined camphor is applied on face twice to clear acne, black spots and leucoderma. Paste of leaf of *Pokasungha* (Ageratum conyzoides) mixed with turmeric is given to children to cure all types of skin diseases. A piece of clean cloth dipped in latex of *Arakha* (Calotropis gigantea) is dried and burnt; the ash along with mustard oil is applied for scabies, itches, morpion and all types of skin diseases. Unripe fruit paste of *Kaniyari* (Cascabela thevetia) is also applied on itches and abscess. Latex of *Agara* (Argemone mexicana) is very effective on herpes, scabies, eczema, angular stomatitis, during conjunctivitis, opthalmia and eye burning. One teaspoon of rhizome powder of *Taltmuli* (Curculigo orchioides) is taken with warm water twice a day in empty stomach for all types of skin disorders. Seed oil of *Dimbiri* (Ficus racemosa) and lime is mixed thoroughly in a brass container until it becomes yellow and it is applied on eczema.[29]

Leaves of *Basanga* (Justicia adhatoda) boiled in water and then cooled is taken as a medicinal bath for children for preventing skin disease. The bark paste of *Kumbhi* (Careya arborea) is taken orally in skin disease. The seed paste or powder of *Chakunda* (Cassia tora) is also applied on various skin diseases. Leaf paste of *Anasorisa* (Cleome gynandra) is very effective to get cured from various types of skin diseases. Rhizome paste of *Haldi* (Curcuma longa) is taken orally and applied externally to prevent skin irritation. Paste prepared from bark powder of *Babulla* (Acacia nilotica) is also applied on skin to check irritation. Leaf juice of *Indramarisa* (Acalypha indica) is applied on affected portions to cure scabies. The juice of the leaf of *Apamaranga* (Achyranthes aspera) is prescribed to cure boil and skin eruptions. Root and bark paste of *Ankula* (Alangium salvifolium) is also used in case of skin eruption. Besides this, paste of leaf of *Bhuinimba* (Andrographis paniculata) along with turmeric is used in case of skin diseases like scabies, eczema etc. Fresh root of *Agara* (Argemone mexicana) is eaten 2 to 3 times daily to reduce fever and to cure skin diseases. Juice of leaf along with common salt is also applied particularly on skin itching. Latex of *Agara* (Argemone mexicana) is also applied on the affected skin to cure dropsy. Decoction of bark and leaf of *Nimba* (Azadirachta indica) is very effective in case of skin diseases.[30]

Poultice of fresh young leaves of *Siali* (Bauhinia vahlii) is anointed on skin to get soothing effect during skin irritation. Paste of thorns of *Simili* (Bombax ceiba) mixed with turmeric is applied on boils for quick burst. Juice of leaves of *Chakunda* (Cassia tora) is used to cure skin eruptions.[31]

Leaves of *Bhuinimba* (Andrographis paniculata) are crushed with *Haldi* (Curcuma longa) and applied on itches and in other skin infections. Bark paste of *Modimodia phal* (Helicteres isora) is considered to be a remedy for scabies. The whole plant of *Pitasaga* (Glinus oppositifolius) is dried and crushed to make a paste and anointed on wounds, scabies and different skin diseases. The whole plant of *Bhuinamla* (Phyllanthus fraternus) is crushed to paste and applied externally to cure scabies, herpes and other skin diseases.[32] The plant *Ambiliti* (Cayratia trifolia) is ground with seeds of *Banasorisa* (Cleome viscosa) and the content is warmed up and then anointed over affected parts to cure skin disease.[33]

In case of allergy, they apply the paste of *Karanja* (Pongamia pinnata) leaves along with *Haldi* (Curcuma longa). The whole plant of *Paunsia* (Aerva lanata) is dried and crushed to paste and applied on herpes.[34]

Scalds and Burns

Ash of the flower of *Kantasido* (Leonotis nepetifolia) is made into paste and applied to scalds and burns.[35] Paste of *Gandha Tulsi* (Ogratissimum) along with juice of *Bisalyakarani* (Tridax procumbens) is applied to heal burns. The jell of *Gheekuanri* (Aloe Vera) helps for quick healing in case of burn injury.[36]

Asthma

Dry leaves of *Apamarangaa* (Achyranthes aspera) are smoked to relieve asthma. Leaves of *Basanga* (Justicia adhatoda) are burnt and the smoke is inhaled to cure asthma. Leaf juice of *Puruni* (Boerhavia diffusa) is taken orally by patients suffering from asthma. Asthma may be kept under check if 1 gm. of seeds of *Chakunda* (Cassia tora) is crushed and boiled in a cup of water and taken twice a day. The aqueous extract of the root of *Tirkatia*

(Clerodendrum serratum) is given for cure of asthma, cough and cold. Flowers of *Arakha* (Calotropis gigantea) are fried in cow ghee and one flower each time is taken twice a day for 30 days to get relieved from asthma. *Haldi* (Curcuma longa) powder mixed with sugar-cane molasses and mustard oil is also taken orally to relieve asthma. Decoction of the fruit *Harida* (Terminalia chebula) is used to cure asthma. Flowers of *Ankranti* (Solanum xanthocarpum) fried in ghee are chewed every day for 15 days to cure cough and asthma.[37]

Besides, root bark decoction of *Basanga* (Justicia adhatoda) with honey is taken orally in empty stomach to cure asthma.[38] Decoction of *Indramarisa* (Acalypha indica) is also effective for patients suffering from asthma and bronchitis. It is taken twice a day till the disease is controlled.[39] Decoction of bark of *Asadua* (Capparis zeylanica) is administered thrice daily to cure cough, asthma and throat inflammations.[40]

Headache

The Kondhs term for headache is *Kapadabisa*. They use some herbal medicines in case of repeated occurrence of severe headache. The juice of *Begunia* (Vitex negundo) leaves if anointed on the forehead heals headache. Seeds of *Bichhuati* (Laporpea interrupta) are also applied as a substitute medicine. But it gives a burning sensation for sometime.[41]

Latex of *Arakha* (Calotropis gigantean) is also applied on forehead to get relief from migraine and headache. Decoction of seed powder of the plant *Bidanga* (Embelia ribes) and *Dhania* (Coriandrum sativum) (50 gm each) along with two tea spoon of honey is taken in empty stomach early morning and evening for 15 to 20 days to cure headache, migraine and dizziness. One to two drops of leaf juice of *Gayasa* (Leucas aspera) is poured in one of the nostrils to cure migraine and headache.

Leaf paste of *Lajakulilata* (Mimosa pudica) is anointed on forehead to get relief from headache and migraine. Leaf juice of *Gangasiuli* (Nyctanthes arbor-tristis) is poured into the nostrils twice a day to cure sinusitis, headache and nasal bleeding. Stem powder of *Guluchi* (Tinospora cordifolia) with equal amount of honey is taken in empty stomach twice daily to cure headache and migraine.[42] Paste of fresh leaf of *Jhanjika* (Breynia rhamnoides) is applied on head for cooling effect during headache and head reeling. Bark of *Sunari* (Cassia fistula) is pounded and also anointed in the fore head to cure headache.[43]

Throat Infections

Dried leaves of *Jhanjika* (Breynia rhamnoides) are used as smoke in case of throat irritation and swollen tonsils. Decoction of bark of *Asadua* (Capparis zeylanica) is taken thrice daily to cure cough, asthma and throat inflammations.[44]

Food Poisoning

Decoction of seed of *Kaincha* (Abrus precatorius) is taken orally to clean the stomach during indigestion and food poisoning. The seeds of *Apamaranga* (Achyranthes aspera) are taken with water to induce vomiting in case of indigestion and food poisoning.[45] Powder of dried root and bark of *Simili* (Bombax ceiba) are used to induce vomiting during food poisoning. Powder of dried leaf and shoot of *Asadua* (Capparis zeylanica) is used as a tooth powder to stop toothache. This is also taken with water as an antidote in case of food poisoning.[46]

Dysentery, Diarrhoea and Cholera

Diarrhoea is called *Patadi* and dysentery is called *Neripata* by the Kondhs. Root paste of *Apamaranga* (Achyranthes aspera) is administered during cholera, indigestion and diarrhoea. About 10 gm. leaves of *Hemakedara* (Kalanchoe pinnata) and seven *Golamaricha* (Piper nigrum) are pasted and taken with water to cure diarrhoea and dysentery. About 100 gm. bark juice of *Kumbhi* (Careya arborea) with raw cow milk is also administered to cure dysentery. Leaf juice of *Duba* (Cynodon dactylon) with sugar candy is prescribed to small kids to cure diarrhoea and vomiting. Juice of *Mukhamali* flower (Tagetes erecta) is given in empty stomach to cure dysentery. Stem bark paste prepared from plant *Dimbiri* (Ficus racemosa) in mother's milk is given to small kids to cure diarrhoea and indigestion. Paste prepared with about 10 gm. root of *Sugandhi* (Hemidesmus indicus) with 2/3 *Golamaricha* (Piper nigrum) is taken in three doses daily to cure diarrhoea of babies. Seed paste of *Keruan* (Holarrhena pubescens) is given with water for curing stomachache and diarrhoea. Decoction of equal amount of bark of *Mahula* (Madhuca indica), *Amba (*Mangifera indica) and *Jamukoli (*Syzygium cumini) with honey is taken daily for 4 to 5 days to cure dysentery and diarrhoea. Root powder of *Bhuinamla* (Phyllanthus fraternus) with Golamaricha (Piper nigrum) is taken with water to cure amoebic dysentery and diarrhoea of children. Paste of tender twigs of *Pijuli* (Psidium guajava) is given with cold water in empty stomach thrice daily to cure blood dysentery.

Young fruit paste of *Dalimba* (Punica granatum) is given orally with water to cure diarrhoea and dysentery. Flower paste of *Vuin Kadamba* (Sphaeranthus indicus) is given in empty stomach to cure dysentery, diarrhoea and indigestion.[47]

Flowers of *Bela* (Aegle marmelos) are taken for combating vomiting and dysentery. Unripe fruit is taken orally for diarrhoea and dysentery. Pulp of ripe fruit is taken as an effective remedy for dysentery. But in case of blood dysentery, the juice of the root of *Satabari* (Asparagus racemosus) is taken with milk.[48] Dried powder of *Harida* (Terminalia chebula) is taken with water to cure chronic diarrhoea and dysentery. Powder of *Methi* (Trigonella foenum-graecum) is taken with water to cure colic, dysentery and diarrhoea.[49]

Powder of dried unriped fruits of *Bela* (Aegle marmelos) is also taken with water twice daily on empty stomach to cure chronic dysentery. Extract of fresh root of *Satabari* (Asparagus racemosus) boiled with milk and taken orally to cure blood dysentery. Decoction of bark of *Barada* (Bauhinia purpurea) is taken 3 to 4 times daily to cure diarrhoea.[50] Powder of dried gum of *Simili* (Bombax ceiba) is taken with water in empty stomach to stop bleeding during blood dysentery. Young leaves of *Jhanjika* (Breynia rhamnoides) are ground to paste and taken orally with sugar candy to cure diarrhoea. It is taken once a day till cure. Powder of dried gum of *Palash* (Butea monosperma) is taken with water to cure diarrhoea and dysentery. This is taken two times in empty stomach. Raw leaf extraction is taken orally twice a day to cure diarrhoea. Paste of root of *Arakha* (Calotropis gigantean) and bark is taken to cure diarrhoea. Decoction of bark of *Tuthudikanta* (Canthium parviflorum) and young shoot is also given to cure dysentery and diarrhoea. This is taken twice daily till cure.[51]

Fruit paste of *Modimodia phal* (Helicteres isora) is administered for chronic dysentery. Root paste of *Sugandhi* (Hemidesmus indicus) is given with fresh cold milk to infants for dysentery and diarrhoea. Decoction of leaves of *Bhuinamla* (Phyllanthus fraternus) is administered orally in early morning to cure amoebas (amoebic dysentery). Decoction of bark of *Chitaparu* (Plumbago zeylanica) is administered orally to cure dysentery.[52]

Vomiting

In Kondh language vomiting is *Schekanti.* They believe that vomiting is caused by the possession of an evil spirit, indigestion, stomach trouble, poison intake, excessive drinking and morning sickness. When vomiting is caused by possession of an evil spirit 'blowing and whiffing' is resorted to. This is their traditional method of treatment and a *Beju* or *Bejuni* is summoned for the purpose. Vomiting when caused by indigestion salt water is given to the patient. Lemon juice is mixed with it whenever available. When vomiting is caused by stomach trouble *Kunduri* (Coccinia Grandis) leaf juice is orally administered. Excessive drunk person when needs immediate vomiting, old *Tentuli* (Tamarindus indica) preserved for 2 to 3 years is kneaded with water and the liquid is orally administered.[53]

Leaf juice of *Pokasungha* (Ageratum conyzoides), fresh leaf juice of *Mutha* (Cyperus rotundus) mixed with small amount of sugar candy is taken in case of vomiting and diarrhoea.[54] Juice of the paste of fruit of *Amla* (Phyllanthus emblica) mixed with sandal paste and honey is taken to stop vomiting.[55] Crushed fruit juice of *Asadua* (Capparis zeylanica) is taken to reduce bile vomiting.[56]

Stomach Disease

Stomach pain is called *Patobish* by the Kondhs. The roots of *Patalagaruda* (Rauvolfia serpentia) are pounded and the juice is squeezed and heated to lukewarm. About half a cup of this mixture is orally administered daily in an empty stomach till the patient is cured.[57]

One tea spoon of *Mutha* (Cyperus rotundus) dried rhizome powder is taken every day to cure acidity and other stomach diseases. Finely paste of *Mayurachulia* (Elephantopus scaber) root is taken with salt in empty stomach in the morning for 21 days to cure chronic abdomen and stomach pain. Root paste of *Kantei Koli* (Firmiana indica) is taken orally daily with water in empty stomach for 10 to 15 days to cure chronic abdomen pain. A small root piece of *Sugandhi* (Hemidesmus indicus) with seven grains of rice and a little turmeric powder is tied around right hand with the help of seven thread pieces to cure stomachache. Root powder of *Kulthia* (Tephrosia purpurea) with *Golamaricha* (Piper nigrum) powder is taken in empty stomach for stomachache and stomach disorders. [58]

About 20 gm. root of *Sugandhi* (Hemidesmus indicus) is powdered and prescribed twice daily in empty stomach for 21 days for treating indigestion, stomach disorder and acidity. Leaf paste of *Lajakulilata* (Mimosa pudica) with honey is prescribed twice a day in empty stomach for 3/4 days for stomachache and intestinal worms.[59]

Decoction of dried unripe fruit of *Bela* (Aegle marmelos) is taken to check ulceration in the stomach. Raw leaves of *Bela* (Aegle marmelos) are directly chewed to increase the digestive capacity.[60]

Decoction of bark of *Ankula* (Alangium salvifolium) is taken twice daily preferably in empty stomach for constipation. Decoction of root and bark of the same plant is also taken at bed time to expel the worms from intestine. The root juice of *Satabari* (Asparagus racemosus) is taken for hyper acidity and even for peptic ulcer. It is taken 2 to 3 times in a day in empty stomach.[61]

Fresh sap of *Salopa* (Caryota urens) is taken early morning in empty stomach to remove constipation. Poultice of fruit of *Sunari* (Cassia fistula) taken with water to prevent constipation. Decoction of leaves of *Chakunda* (Cassia tora) is taken during constipation to get good results. Decoction of root of *Kerenda koli* (Carissa carandas) is taken to check stomach pain and also used for deworming. Decoction of root of *Akanabindi* (Cissampelos pareira) is taken orally to cure stomach pain and indigestion.[62]

Urine Infection

The paste of root of *Satabari* (Asparagus racemosus) mixed with boiled cow milk is taken for 7 to 10 days to cure urinary infection and burning sensation of the urinary tract. Juice of leaves of *Palash* (Butea monosperma) is taken orally to prevent burning during urination. This is taken two times daily for 2 to 3 months or more.[63]

Typhoid

About 10 gm. leaf of *Apamaranga* (Achyranthes aspera) with seven *Golamaricha* (Piper nigrum) seeds is ground and small tablets of about 2 gm. are made and are taken with water for seven days to cure bilious fever and typhoid.[64]

Leaf paste of *Gayasa* (Leucas aspera) in milk with honey is taken thrice daily for seven days to cure typhoid. Root paste of *Kulthia* (Tephrosia purpurea) with raw milk is taken in empty stomach twice daily for seven days to cure cold fever and typhoid.[65]

Rheumatism

In rheumatism fever, paste of leaves and roots of *Apamaranga* (Achyranthes aspera) along with *Golamaricha* (Piper nigrum) is administered. Paste prepared from 10 gm. of root of *Bela* (Aegle marmelos) and 21 *Golamaricha* (Piper nigrum) is taken with raw milk in empty stomach twice daily for 21 days to cure rheumatism and rheumatic inflammation. One teaspoon of decoction of *Bhuinimba* (Andrographis paniculata) with one teaspoon of honey is taken twice a day in empty stomach for 15 days to cure rheumatic fever. Stem bark paste of *Masania* (Aporusa octandra) is also applied for curing rheumatism.[66]

Two to three teaspoons full of decoction of *Taltmuli* (Curculigo orchiodes) is taken with one teaspoon of honey in empty stomach for 21 to 30 days to cure kidney stone and rheumatic fever. Plant decoction of *Basanga* (Justicia adhatoda) with honey is taken twice daily in empty stomach to cure cold fever and rheumatic fever.[67]

Paste of fresh root bark of *Gandhana* (Premna latifolia) with *Golamaricha* (Piper nigrum) is taken twice daily in empty stomach for 15 days to get relief from rheumatism, body ache and muscle pain. Fomentation of leaf paste also gives relief from rheumatism, sprain and body ache. Root juice of *Patalagaruda* (Rauvolfia serpentina) with water is taken orally to cure body ache and rheumatism. Decoction of stem barks of Kalo plant (Ricinus communis), *Hadabhanga* (Cissus quadrangulis) and *Nirgundi* (Vitex negundo) leaves is fomented on the affected area for rheumatic swelling and arthritis. To cure arthritis, rheumatism and inflammation, one teaspoon of stem decoction of *Guluchi* (Tinospora cordifolia) with half teaspoon honey is taken in empty stomach for one month. Stem decoction with sesame oil is applied on body to get relief from rheumatism, body pain and inflammation. Root decoction of *Nirgundi* (Vitex negundo) is prescribed twice a day in empty stomach to cure rheumatism.[68]

Leaf poultice of *Ankula* (Alangium salvifolium) is applied on joints to get relief from the rheumatic pain. Poultice of root of *Asadua* (Capparis zeylanica) is applied on joints to get relief from rheumatic pain. Decoction of fruit of *Sunari* (Cassia fistula) is taken to reduce rheumatic pain.[69] Poultice of leaf of *Bheru* (Chloroxylon swietiana) is applied on joints to reduce rheumatic pain.[70] Leaf pastes of *Brahmi* (Bocopa monnieri) mixed with petroleum is applied on rheumatism.[71]

Ear Pain and Ear Infection

The extracted juice of *Salap* (Caryota urens) root is heated to lukewarm and put in the ear. Heated *Arakha* (Calotropis gigantea) leaves are pounded and the juice is squeezed in the infected ear of the patient.[72] Lukewarm leaf juice of *Arakha* (Calotropis gigantea) is used as ear drops to relieve earache.[73]

Two to three drops of juice of the leaves of *Banatulasi* (Ocimum gratissimum) are put in the ear in case of severe pain in the ear drum, loss of audible capacity, discharge and pus.[74] The decoction of the leaves of *Indramaris* (Acalypha indica) is used for ear pain.[75]

Hysteria

The young and the adolescent are mostly affected by this disease. The belief is that the disease is caused by spirit intrusion; still they use medicines for it.

Decoction of roots and leaves of *Tuthudi kanta* (Canthium parviflorum) is taken in case of hysteria.[76] Infusion of flowers of *Sebati* (Chrysanthemum coronarium) is prescribed for hysteria.[77]

Eye Pain and Eye Infection

One or two drops of onion juice are applied to eradicate eye infection. The affected eye is also frequently dabbed with a piece of cloth soaked in turmeric water.[78] Latex of *Odisamari* or *Agara* (Argemone mexicana) is applied during conjunctivitis, and eye burning. Leaf juice of *Odisamari* (Argemone maxicana) is also applied on eye corners in the morning and before bed to cure eye inflammation and conjunctivitis. Purple flower juice (4/5 drops) of *Aparajita* (Cliteria tarnatea) is poured directly into the eye to cure conjunctivitis and eye pain. Leaf juice with little rock salt is also applied to the eye to get relief from eye swelling and blurred disease.[79]

Latex of the plant of *Agara* (Argemone mexicana) is applied on the corners of the eye at bed time to cure eye inflammations.[80] Juice of the stem of *Jhanjika* (Breynia rhamnoides) is directly applied on eyes to cure conjunctivitis. This is repeated 2 to 3 times in a day till complete cure.[81]

Mouth Infection

Paste of 20 gm. root of *Kharakhari* (Elephantopus scaber) with seven *Golamaricha* (Piper nigrum) is prescribed to cure mumps and mouth ulcers. One tea spoon root powder of *Sugandhi* (Hemidesmus indicus) with honey is prescribed for 3 to 4 days to small kids to cure mouth infections and herpes. Raw leafs of *Vuin Kadamba* (Sphaeranthus indicus) are chewed or leaf juice is administered orally during mouth ulcer and other mouth diseases.[82]

Decoction of leaves of *Kadamba* (Neolamarckia cadamba) is used as mouth wash to cure ulceration in mouth. This is performed 3 to 4 times in a day.[83]

Toothache

Seeds of *Bhejibaigana* or *Ankranti* (Solanum xanthocarpum) mixed with castor oil is put on a hot iron dish and the smoke is inhaled by the patient. They also apply *Arakha* (Calotropis gigantea) latex on the affected teeth. *Dimbiri* (*Ficus racemosa*) latex is also applied as a substitute for this.[84]

Stem of *Babulla* (Acacia nilotica) is used as tooth brush to strengthen the gums. Few raw leaves of *Dantarikanta* (Acacia pennata) are chewed along with sugar and *Jeera* (Cuminum cyminum) to stop bleeding of the gums. The process is continued till the bleeding stops.[85] A piece of root of *Apamaranga* (Achyranthes aspera) is crushed and chewed to cure tooth ache. Fresh leaves of *Nimba* (Azadirachta indica) are chewed to check gum infections.[86] Powder of dried root and bark of *Siriso* (Albizia lebbeck) is used as a tooth powder for strengthening the gums.[87]

Sprain

The Dongria Kondhs apply lukewarm turmeric paste fried with castor oil on the area of sprain for 3 to 4 times in a day till cure. The heated paste of *Bisalyakarani* (Tridax procumbens) is applied in case of sprain.[88] The tender branches of *Baigaba* (Jatropha curcas) are put on live charcoal and twisted to extract the fluid. The fluid oozing branches are pressed over the affected part of the body.[89]

Fracture

Tender part of *Hada Bhanga* (Cissus quadrangula) bush and black gram are grinded to paste and applied evenly on the fractured portion in case of fracture.[90] Stem bark paste of *Masania* (Aporosa octandra) is plastered on the bone-fractured area with the help of cloth for one month. In bone crack and bone fracture, a coating of castor oil is applied on the area and then plastered with the paste of stem of the of *Hadabhanga* (Cissus quadrangula) plant and cloth.[91] Paste of fresh bark of *Kumbhi* (Careya arborea) mixed with unboiled milk (Cow/Goat) is applied on the fractured limbs. It is tied with the help of bamboo sticks and rope and kept for a week. This process is repeated for 3 to 4 weeks.[92]

On severe external injury, the leaves of *Bilati Sido* (Pedilanthus tithymalodes) are directly pasted after warming applied on the affected area as plasters. The whole plant of *Bisiripi* (Sida cordifolia) is boiled and crushed to a paste and applied on fractures and swellings. The fracture part is often tightened with the support of bamboo sticks and left for about 2 to 3 months.[93]

They apply the paste of *Hadabhanga* (Cissus quadrangula) barks, *Sunari* (Cassia fistual) leaves and *Golamaricha* (Piper nigrum) on the fracture area for seven days to set it.[94]

Cuts and Wounds

Frequent incidents of minor and major accidental cuts are reported in Kondh villages, which result in heavy bleeding. To stop bleeding and to heal such wounds they use different herbal medicines. This stops bleeding immediately and also lessens the pain. For healing the wound the Kondhs anoint the juice of *Bisalyakarani* (Tridex procumbens). Warm turmeric paste is also applied on the injury which gives quick relief. The root of *Apamaranga* (Achyranthes aspera) is fried in castor oil and tide on the cuts and wounds with the help of a cloth for healing. Leaf juice of *Pokasungha* (Ageratum conyzoides) is applied to cure abscess, itches, cuts and wounds for checking bleeding and healing. Leaf paste of *Sitaphala* (Annona squamosa) is applied on wounds to disinfect the area. Stem bark paste of *Masania* (Aporosa octandra) is used for healing up of cuts, wounds and itches. Stem bark decoction of *Dimbiri* (Ficus racemosa) is used for healing quickly of cuts and wounds. Root paste of *Keruan* (Holarrhena pubescens) is also applied on cut and wound.[95]

Bark powder of *Ashoka* (Saraca asoca) or leaf juice of *Bisalyakarani* (Tridax procumbens) or dried rhizome of *Amla* (Phyllanthus emblica) is applied externally after any physical injury to stop bleeding.[96]

Decoction of *Bhuinimba* (Andrographis paniculata) is used for washing septic wounds and boils. Poultice of bark of *Phansi* (Anogeissus acuminate) is applied on the cuts and wounds to check bleeding.[97] Latex of *Arakha* (Calotropis gigantea) is applied directly on the cuts for early healing. Paste of young leaves and shoots of *Asadua* (Capparis zeylanica) is applied on boils to get relief.[98] Juice of crushed leaves of *Bheru* (Chloroxylon swietiana), are directly applied on the cuts and wounds.[99]

Stem juice of *Amari* (Ipomoea carnea) along with dust is used as antiseptic to small cuts. Stem juice is also applied externally to alleviate pain on external injuries. Paste of *Chitaparu* (Plumbago zeylanica) is applied to the wound and also taken orally for immediate cure.[100]

Root paste of *Langalangalia Kanda* (Glorsa superba) is applied for five days on the cut and wound by iron or glass.[101] Coconut coir is burnt and the ash is made paste with coconut oil. This paste is anointed upon the sore which heals it slowly.[102]

Ring Worms

Leaf juice of *Apamaranga* (Achyranthes aspera) with salt is applied on ringworms. Seed oil of *Agara* (Argemone mexicana) is applied on itches and ringworm.[103] In some cases, juice of *Agara* (Argemone mexicana) along with common salt is applied particularly on ringworm.[104] In case of ringworm the affected area is scraped with a clean dry stone or wood and when it emits blood or fluid the milk of unripe fruit *Amrutabhanda* (Carica papaya) is applied. The wound is kept open till it is healed.[105]

Worms

Poultice of root of *Tuthudi kanta* (Canthium parviflorum) is taken with water in empty stomach at morning to remove worms from intestine.[106] Seeds of *Chakunda* (Cassia tora) are crushed and taken with water at bed time to remove thread worms.[107] Decoction of leaves or leaf paste of *Bhuinnima* (Andrographis paniculata) taken orally before bed against round worm.[108] An admixture of turmeric and *Nimba* (Azadirachta indica) paste is taken orally by the patient once daily before food in case of worm infestation.[109]

Gastric

One teaspoonful leaf powder of *Bela* (Aegle marmelos) is taken orally in empty stomach for 15 to 30 days to cure gastric problems. Young fruit boiled in raw milk with seven *Golamaricha* (Piper nigrum) is taken in empty stomach to cure gastro-exophageal reflux.[110]

Leaf juice of *Taltmuli* (Curculigo orchioides) with a little amount of honey is prescribed for intestinal worms, indigestion and gastric ulcer and stomach disorders of children. Tablets made from paste of rhizome of *Karalakanta* (Dolichandnone falcata) and seven *Golamaricha* (Piper nigrum) are taken with warm water (two at a time), twice a day in empty stomach for 21 days to cure gastro-esophageal reflux. Seed decoction of *Bidanga* (Embelia ribes) with honey is also taken in empty stomach twice daily for 15 days to cure gastric, bile and lumbago (stabbing backache). Leaf juice of *Gayasa* (Leucas aspera) along with honey is taken twice a day to cure rheumatism, intermittent fever, cough, asthma, fistula and gastric disorder. Young leaf juice of *Amba* (Mangifera indica) and *Pijuli* (Psidium guajava) with *Golamaricha* (Piper nigrum) powder and raw cow milk is taken twice a day in empty stomach to cure vomiting, gastric disorder, bile and acidity.[111] Powder of dried root of *Barada* (Bauhinia purpurea) is taken with water to remove wind from stomach during gastritis.[112]

Acidity

Two to three fruits of *Bidanga* (Embelia ribes) are chewed in case of acidity.[113]About six grams of raw stem bark of *Kochila* (Strychnos nuxvomica) is ground with twenty-one *Golamaricha* (Piper nigrum) and made into tablet size, dried in shade and kept in bottles. Daily one tablet is taken for seven days to cure excess acidity. The root juice of Satabari (Asparagus racemosus) is taken for hyper acidity 2 to 3 times in a day in empty stomach.[114]

Fresh leaves of *Bela* (Aegle marmelos) is taken early in the morning in empty stomach to avoid acidity, discomfort or pain in the stomach.[115]

Insomnia

Fried leaves of *Sunusunia* (Marsilea minuta) are taken with food to cure insomnia.[116] For sleeplessness, *Lajakuli* (Mimosa pudica) juice is orally administered. The Kondhs also believe that if a part of the creeper is kept on the bed it induces sleep.[117]

Jaundice

The Kondhs believe that seven *mantra* salt if chewed then the patient suffering from jaundice is cured. Besides this they use juice from *Kaincha* (Abrus precatorius) root as another substitute for this disease.[118]

Seven leaves of the plant *Pedhipedhica* (Abutilon indicum) with seven *Golamaricha* (Piper nigrum) seeds are ground and the paste is mixed with one glass of raw milk or with sugar candy (*Misry*) powder and are taken orally in empty stomach for seven days (daily twice) to cure jaundice. Root sap of *Dimbiri* (Ficus racemosa) with sugar candy powder is taken twice a day in empty stomach to cure jaundice. Plant decoction of *Basanga* (Justicia adhatoda) with honey is taken in empty stomach twice daily for seven days to cure jaundice. Root paste of *Manjuati* (Lawsonia inermis) with *Golamaricha* (Piper nigrum) or *Dimbiri* (Ficus racemosa) fruit juice is taken with cold water in empty stomach to cure jaundice. Lime coat applied on a completely ripen banana and kept in open field over night is given next day early morning in empty stomach for seven days to cure jaundice. Decoction of stem bark of *Salo* (Shorea robusta) plant along with *Ankula (*Alangium salvifolium) roots, *Mahul* (Madhuca indica) root bark and *Jamokoli (*Syzygium cumini) stem bark is taken in the morning in empty stomach for 21 days to cure jaundice.[119]

Fruit powder of *Harida* (Terminalia chebula), *Bahada* (Terminalia bellirica) added with the juice of *Amla* (Phylanthus embelica) is taken twice daily in empty stomach for one month to cure jaundice.[120] Root decoction (50 ml.) of *Saptaphena* (Opuntia stricta) root (10 gm.), 20 gm. *Sunthi* (Zangibar officinale)) seven *Golamaricha* (Piper nigrum), 3 to 5 small cardamoms and 10 gm. *Kalajeera* (Nigella sativa) are mixed and given twice daily for seven days to cure jaundice.[121]

Nightblindness

The leaves of *Satabari* (Asparagus racemosus) fried with ghee is taken twice in a week for about one month to cure night-blindness. Powder of dried gums of *Sirisa* (Albizia lebbeck) is taken with water to prevent and cure night blindness.[122]

Constipation

Seeds of *Sirisa* (Albizia lebbeck) plants powdered and a pinch of the powder taken continuously for seven days cures constipation. Juice of *Mutha* (Cyperus rotundus) plant is given three times a day for three days to cure constipation.[123] Leaves of *Indramarisha* (Acalypha indica) is made thick paste and applied at anus to cure constipation.[124] Juice of the *Brahmi* (Bacopa monnieri) plant is taken to get rid of constipation.[125] Juice of the leaves of *Thalakudi* (Centella asiatica) taken with raw-milk of cow to get rid of constipation.[126]

Fissure

Paste of about 10 gm. adventitious roots of *Bara* (Ficus benghalensis) with 3/4 *Labanga* (Syzygium aromaticum) is taken either with a cup of *Satabari* (Asparagus racemosus) rhizome juice or *Bara* (Ficus benghalensis) bark juice in empty stomach twice a day for 3 to 4 weeks to cure fissure. Paste of stem bark (10 gm.) of *Keruan* (Holarrhena pubescens) and 21 *Golamaricha* (Piper nigrum) seeds is given in empty stomach twice daily for 21 days with cool water or raw milk to cure fissure. Cakes of equal size prepared from paste of seven leaves of *Baruna* (Crateva magna) with 150 gm. wet rice are taken thrice daily to cure fissure.[127]

Leprosy

Bhramaramari (Antiria toxicaria) tree, a rare availability is the only recognized medicine found by the medicine man, who uses its roots to cure leprosy. This tree is found in the dense forest upon the rocky places.[128]

Paste of roots of *Apamarangaa* (Achyranthes aspera) with cow urine is applied on leprosy wound daily 2/3 times for one month for cure. Paste of about 20 gm. seed of *Chakunda* (Cassia tora) with cow urine is applied on leprosy wounds daily twice for one month. Watering juice of the root of *Guluchi* (Tinospora cordifolia) is applied on leprosy affected parts of the body[129] Poultice of bark and leaf of *Mahanimba* (Melia azedarach) is applied externally in case of leprosy. It is also taken orally for months together to get good results.[130] Poultice of root of *Dhala Chitaparu* (Plumbago zeylanica) is applied externally to get good results in leprosy.[131] Tuber paste of the plant *Gowsingo* (Colocasia esculenta) is mixed with caster oil and applied locally to cure leprosy wounds.[132]

Snake Bite

Haldi (Curuma longa) and *Patalgaruda* (Rauvolfia serpentina) roots are grinded to paste and anointed upon the spot of bite. The extracted juice from the same is also orally administered.[133] *Gada* (Zingiber zerumbet) root is one effective substitute for snakebite. The extracted juice from the root is orally administered and at the same time a piece of the root is also inhaled by the person.[134]

Juice of leaves of *Banatulasi* (Ocimum gratissimum) is taken for snake bite. Juice of bark of *Dantarikanta* (Acacia pennata) is taken orally as an antidote for snake bite. Leaf and stem paste of *Madaranga* (Alternanthera sessilis) is applied externally on snake bite to reduce pain.[135]

Paste of leaf and bark of *Nimba* (Azadirachta indica) is applied on scorpion stings and snake bite. Flower and fruit paste of *Simili* (Bombax ceiba) is applied in snake bites as an antidote.[136]

Paste of *Ankula* bark (Alngium salvifolium) is applied and administered orally (10 gm.) for snake bite.[137]A finger long root of *Bela* (Aegle marmelos) is ground and made into paste. The paste is taken orally and a little of it is applied on eye lids and the patient is kept awake.[138]

Scorpion and Insect Bite

A piece of root of *Patalagaruda* (Rauvolfia serpentina) is rubbed on a stone and then applied on the wound and also taken orally after dilution against scorpion sting.[139]

Salt and *Haldi* (Curuma longa) paste is anointed over the affected spot. For other insect-bites the affected portion is given a heat fomentation.[140]

Root paste of *Guluchi* (Tinospora cordifolia) is applied in scorpion sting. Decoction of *Arjun* (Terminalia arjuna) bark is an antidote to poison. Gum of *Sal* (Shorea robusta) fried with ghee is applied in scorpion sting. The root paste of *Krushna Kedar* (Globba bulbifera) is applied for scorpion bite. The bark paste and seed paste of *Jamukoli* (Syzygium cumini) is used as an antidote for snake or scorpion bite.[141]

Leaf juice of *Phansi* (Anogeissus acuminate) is applied on the spot of scorpion sting to relief pain.[142]

Bleeding from Nose

Dry cow dung is burnt and its smoke is inhaled by the patient.[143] The leaf juice of *Neelgiri* (Eucaliptus citriodora) is taken orally and raw cow dung is inhaled.[144] Kondhs also believe that this disease is caused by sprit intrusion. Still they take the juice of *Patalgaruda* (Rauvolfia serpentina) plant to stop bleeding from nose.[145]

To Check Bleeding in Case of Injury

In fatal injuries, the stem of *Baunsa* (Bambusa tulda) is crushed to paste and applied along with salvia in the affected area to stop excessive bleeding. This also acts as an antiseptic.[146]

Diabetes

About 20 gm. bark decoction of *Simili* (Bombax ceiba) with one tea spoon turmeric powder is taken twice a day in empty stomach for one month to cure diabetes. Decoction of roots of *Basanga* (Justicia adhatoda), *Akanabindhi* (Cissampelos pareira) root and fruits of *Harida* (Terminalia chebula), *Bahada* (Terminalia bellirica) and *Amla* (Phyllanthus emblica) with one drop of cow ghee is taken orally thrice a day for one month in empty stomach to cure diabetes. Decoction of fresh leaves of *Kalara* (Momordica charantia), *Gudamari* (Gymnema sylvestre) and fruits of *Amla (*Phyllanthus emblica) with one teaspoon of honey is taken twice daily in empty stomach for one month to cure diabetes.[147]

Fleshy part, external to the seed of *Harida* (Terminalia chebula) and seeds of *Jamukoli* (Syzygum cumini) are collected and left for drying under a *Kalara* (Momordica charantia) plant. Then the seeds are taken in equal quantities and pasted. Small tablets are made out of it. Two tablets a day controls diabetes.[148]

The barks of *Nimba* (Azadirachra indica) and *Karanja* (Pongamia pinnata) are boiled together and taken regularly to cure diabetes.[149]

Leaves of *Bhuinimba* (Andrographis paniculata) consumed for curing diabetes. The leaves and seeds of *Bhuinamla* (Phyllanthus fraternus) are used as decoction for diabetes.[150]

Paralysis

The root paste of *Sajana* (Moringa oleifera) mixed with salt is applied on paralytic part of the body to get good results.[151] The milky juice of *Lohasiju* (Euphorbia antiquorum) is also used to cure paralysis.[152]

A poultice of leaves of *Sunari* (Cassia fistula) is taken orally in facial paralysis to get good results.[153]

Face Disease

The plant and root ash of *Dhala Aparajita* (Clitoria ternatea) with cow butter is taken orally for one month to clean pimples and facial spots. [154]

Root of *Kaladudura* (Datura metel) is ground with rock salt and gently warmed, then applied on the face of boils and pimples for cure.[155]

Small Pox

In case of small pox, the leaves of *Nimba* (Azadirachta indica) are spread around the bed of the patient. The patient is made to sleep upon *Nimba* (Azadirachta indica) leaves and dried leaves of *Nimba* (Azadirachta indica) are burnt in a pot near the patient to provide soothing smoke. Water boiled with leaves of *Nimba* (Azadirachta indica) is used as a bath to get relief at the time of small pox. *Basanga* (Justicia adhatoda) leaves boiled with water is consumed to prevent small pox. *Methi* (Trigonella foenum-graecum) water is given to the person suffering from small pox, chicken pox and measles. Juice of *Ada* (Zangiber officinale) is taken with juice of *Tulsi* (Ocimum sanctum) for curing small pox.[156]

Bark paste of *Kumbhi* (Careya arborea) is applied externally in small pox. Decoction of bark of *Kumbhi* (Careya arborea) is taken twice daily to reduce fever due to chicken pox and measles.[157]

Body Ache

The decoction of seed of *Bana Kolathia* (Atylosia scarabaeoides) is taken during body ache.[158]

Decoction of *Akanbindi* (Cissampelos pareira) is given to new mothers to reduce body ache. In case of pain in any part of the body, the latex of *Dimiri* (Ficus racemosa) and salt are mixed into a paste and applied externally on the affected area directly to alleviate pain. The paste is used as a plaster with the help of a white paper and left for 2 to 3 days to reduce swelling in the body. Fresh rhizomes of *Kakadakanda* (Angiopteris evecta) are pounded after washing and taken orally to cure body ache and leg pain.[159]

Oil from the seeds of *Mahula* (Madhuca indica) along with leaves of *Tila* (Sesamum indicum) is applied on the body of the patient suffering from body ache. It is advised to take bread of *Mahula* flower and *Mahula* beer is applied over the body to get relief from body ache.[160]

Kidney Problem

The *dal* prepared from the seeds of *Bana Kolathia* (Atylosia scarabaeoides) is eaten for preventing kidney stone formation. It is also prescribed as a medicine to get relief from kidney problems.[161]

Raw Onion is taken as medicine to cure kidney and gallstone problems. Seeds of *Dalimba* (Punica granatum) paste mixed with cow milk are recommended for removing kidney stone of the expectant mothers.[162]

Gynecological Diseases

Among the Kondh girls after puberty the menstrual flow continues for 4 to 7 days. Irregularities in this cycle are not considered a disease. Whenever there is excess discharge or the flow continues for more than normal period they consult a medicine man who gives some herbal medicines to check it. The juice extracted from the roots of *Patalagaruda* (Rauvolfia serpentina) is administered orally which helps to cure such disease. Menopause occurs within the age of 45 to 50 years. Those who desire earlier menopause consult a medicine man. Equal quantity of *Karkati* (Momordica disica) and *Patalgaruda* (Rauvolfia serpentina) roots are pounded and the extracted juice is orally administered to the woman who desires earlier menopause. Three years old *Jada* (Ricinus communis) bark, *Kalara* (Momrdica charantia) and *Bajramuli* (Sida acuta) roots are pounded to extract juice. This mixture is orally administered which helps quick falling of placenta. Long preserved red *Padma* (Nelumbo nucifera) is mixed with wheat flour and administered orally also acts as a substitute medicine.[163]

Seeds of *Kaincha* (Abrus precatorius) are taken with molasses after menstruation to prevent conception. Seed of this plant is also used as suppository to induce abortion in case of early pregnancy.

The root paste of *Apamaranga* (Achyranthes aspera) with cold water is given to stop bleeding after abortion. Decoction of root of *Madaranga* (Alternanthera sessilis) is taken twice a day to check excess bleeding during menstruation.[164]

Paste of root of *Satabari* (Asparagus racemosus) is taken during pregnancy to prevent abortion. Decoction of root is also prescribed to the lactating mothers to increase milk secretion. It is taken 2 to 3 times in a week. Boiled roots are directly eaten to cure anemia due to profuse bleeding during menstruation. Crushed roots are taken with milk to rectify infertility among women.[165]

The shoot of *Kadali* (Musa paradisiaca) plant is tied loosely to the neck of the women and kept under observation. The shoot is removed as soon as the placenta comes out. A small root of *Tentuli* (Tamarindus indica) plant is fixed to the ear of the women and she is advised to sleep flat on a mat which helps in delivering the child easily. The post delivered women is advised for licking the latex of the plant *Dhala dudura* (Datura metel) twice a day (morning and evening) for secretion of milk.[166]

A piece of root of *Patalagaruda* (Rauvolfia serpentina) ground with 5/10 *Golamaricha* (Piper nigrum) is diluted with water and taken orally for relief from pain after menstrual cycle. Decoction of *Ashoka* (Saraca asoca) bark is taken with milk prevents miscarriage and frequent still birth. The pregnant woman is advised to smell the root of *Langalangalia kanda* (Gloriosa superba) and to keep some of its root on her hair knot which helps her for easy delivery Root juice of *Saruniali* (Tasminum roxburghianum) extracted and mixed with an equal amount of garlic juice and is given to ladies immediately after delivery as a tonic. Leaves of *Dudhi* (Cryptolepis buchananii) are taken as leafy vegetable during lactation period of women.[167]

A mixture of seed powder of *Ramphal* (Annon reticulate) with *Golamaricha* (Piper nigrum) is given to spoil the pregnancy of 3 to 4 months. Three ml. fresh juice of *Baruna* (Crateva nurvala) mixed with one gm. seed powder of *Golamaricha* (Piper nigrum) is taken by women in the seventh days of menstrual cycle as a contraceptive.[168]

Malaria

Leaf juice of *Gangasiuli* (Nyctanthes arbor-tristis) is given in empty stomach for curing malaria. Leaf of *Gangasiuli* (Nyctanthes arbor-tristis), root of *Bhuinimba* (Andrographis paniculata) and juice of *Tulsi* (Ocimum sanctum) are mixed and taken with *Golamaricha* (Piper nigrum). Besides this, bark of *Nimba* (Azadirachta indica), *Guluchi* (Tinospora cordifolia), *Pitapotal* (Cayratia pedata) and *Chireita* (Andrographis paniculata) are mixed with water and decoction is prepared and taken twice daily to cure malaria. But *Guluchi* (Tinospora cordifolia) and *Nimba* (Azadirachta indica) together boiled in water. The clothes which Kondhs wear regularly are put into it and boiled. If those clothes are put on, it is believed, mosquito will not bite. This is one of the preventive measures for malaria.[169] Juice of seven leaves of *Gangasiuli* (Nyctanthes arbor-tristis) with two teaspoon honey taken daily twice for malaria.[170]

Powder of *Bahada* (Terminalia bellirica), bark of *Aswattha* (Ficus religiosa) and seeds of *Kendu* (Diospyros melanoxylom) are given to the patient thrice daily. Powder of *Nimba* (Azadirachta indica) leaves and seeds along with *Pippali* (Piper longum) are administered to the patient twice daily. Kondhs believe that if one leaf of *Nimba* (Azadirachta indica) is taken continuously for twenty one days excluding Sundays, a person will not suffer from malaria for one year [171]

Dog and Jackal Bite

Root paste of *Apamaranga* (Achyranthes aspera) with *misry* powder is prescribed for 21 days in empty stomach against dog and jackal bite.[172] Bark paste of *Ankula* (Alangium salvifolium) is given to the patient in case of dog and jackal bite. Root paste of *Krushnakedar* (Globba bulbifera) is applied for jackal and dog bite.[173]

Medicine to Induce Complete Barrenness

The Kondhs believe that if seven *Kaincha* (Abrus precatorius) seeds are eaten by a woman, she never conceives. After that *Bonobeto* (Calamus tenuis) is an effective herbal medicine used by the Dongria Kondhs. This root is pounded and the juice is squeezed for the medicine. Oral administration of about half a cup of this juice induces complete barrenness.[174]

Piles

Langalanglia Kanda (Gloriosa superba) root paste is applied by Kondhs on the anus for five days for piles. Cold infusion of *Duba* (Cynodon dactylon) grass is taken orally to stop bleeding from piles. Seed paste of *Kenua* (Holarrhena pubescens) is taken to cure piles. The ash of fruiting spikes of *Apamaranga* (Achyranthes aspera) is applied externally on piles after defecation. Seeds of *Banatulasi* (Ocimum gratissimum) with water are taken daily for about a week to relieve from piles and constipation.[175] Poultice of fresh leaves of *Indramarisa* (Acalypha indica) is directly applied on anus and piles to get a soothing effect. Decoction of bark and seed of *Siriso* (Albizia lebbeck) is taken 2 to 3 times a day to prevent bleeding from piles.[176] Ripe or unripe fruits of *Nimba* (Azadirachta indica) are consumed to cure piles.[177]

A handful leaves of *Barada* (Bauhinia purpurea) is ground with one stand of charming feather of peacock and a little of *Goruchina* to a thick paste. The paste is whipped with a lobe of jaggery and taken orally once. After sometime one egg of a hen is cracked and placed on the anus.[178]

Indigestion

Leave paste of *Prasaruni* (Paederia foetida) is taken with *Golamaricha* (Piper nigrum) for indigestion. Fermented liquor made from the fruits of *Amla* (Phylanthus emblica) is given in indigestion.[179] Leaf juice of *Bhuinimba* (Andrographis paniculata) is taken to increase appetite and to improve digestion.[180]

Decoction of leaves of *Apamaranga* (Achyranthes aspera) is applied to cure indigestion. For indigestion the extract of ripe fruit of *Bela* (Aegle marmelos) with water is given. The tea of garlic, sweetened with honey is recommended for indigestion.[181]

Leucorrhoea

Paste of leaves of *Baila* (Lablab purpureus) and flowers are taken in leucorrhoea. Three ml. decoction of root of *Arakha* (Calotropis gigantea) with paste of *Peppali* (Pipper longum) is given to the women in empty stomach continuously for ten days for the treatment of leucorrhoea. Decoction of the plant *Puruni* (Boerhavia diffusa) is given once a day in the early morning for fifteen days for the treatment of leucorrhoea.[182]

The bark juice of *Arjuna* (Terminalia arjuna) and *Asoka* (Saraca asoca) is taken orally to cure leucorrhoea.[183] The gum of *Babula* (Acacia nilotica) is dissolved in water and the solution is applied on the sex organ to cure leucorrhoea.[184]

Gonorrhea

Plant juice of *Puruni* (Boerhavia diffusa) is considered as an effective medicine for gonorrhea. Underground part of the plant *Taltamuli* (Curculigo orchioides) with root of *Kolathia* (Tephrosia purpurea) is ground and applied to cure gonnorrhoea.[185]

Fits

The paste of *Apamarnga root* (Achyranthes aspera) along with *Baila* (Lablab purpureus) is applied to cure fits.[186]

To Increase Potency

Decoction of seed of *Siali* (Bauhinia vahlii) is taken 2/3 times in a week to increase potency among males. Decoction of root of *Simili* (Bombax ceiba) is taken by males to cure impotency. This is taken 2/3 times in a week for few months.[187]

Decoction of the root *Gosingi* (Phyla nodiflora) (3 ml.) with unboiled egg is given to women to increase potency.[188]

Mental Disorder

Root paste of *Patalagaruda* (Rauvolfia serpentina) is taken either with raw milk or honey in empty stomach twice a day for 21 days to cure mental disorder.[189] The leaf juice of *Bramhi* (Bacopa monnieri) is used to cure mental disorder, nervous disorder and convulsion.[190] About 25 ml. of leaf juice of *Kalara* (Momordica charantia) mixed with honey is taken orally in the morning for about two to three days to cure madness.[191]

Epilepsy

Root paste of young tree of *Sajana* (Moringa oleifera) is applied for epilepsy.[192] Decoction of root of *Patalagaruda* (Rauvolfia serpentina) is also applied to the person suffering from epilepsy.[193]

Enlarged Spleen

Tuberous root of *Talamuli* (Curculigo orchiodes) is rubbed on a stone and kept in a container. Water poured over a piece of red hot iron (mostly of the ploughing rod) is mixed with it and given to patients three times to cure enlarged spleen. Root paste of young tree of *Sajana* (Moringa oleifera) is also applied for spleen.[194]

Fruits of *Kantaikoli* (Firmiana indica) are taken regularly to cure enlarged spleen.[195] The leaf pulp of *Gheekuanri* (Aloe vera) is applied for spleen.[196]

Anemia

About a handful of flowers of *Gayasa* (Leucas aspera) boiled with cow milk, and the cooled content is given to patients for about fifteen days to cure anemia. Decoction of root of *Hatisundha* (Heliotropium indicum) (10 ml.) with honey (2 ml.) is taken as vitamin for iron deficiency of women against anemia during pregnancy period.[197] The powder of dried root of *Sugandhi* (Hemidesmus indicus) is given with milk to cure anemia after delivery.[198]

From the field study undertaken in the villages of different districts of south Odisha, it has been observed that the Kondhs prefer the indigenous method of treatment even though modern medical facilities are there. But they have some related beliefs regarding the administration of their indigenous medicines. They are of the view that indigenous medicines can not alone cure diseases. To increase the therapeutic effect of the medicine the medicine man enchants *mantra* (magical spell), while administering it. Quiet interestingly when we asked, "What is the use of *mantra*?" The reply was, "*Gada pada nua pale kamata bade.*", which means without *mantra* medicine cannot work successfully.

Almost all medicine men have also common faith or belief regarding the mode of preparation, time of preparation and administration of medicine. Medicine men prepare drugs after taking bath. They are also selective about the time of collection of drug materials. Some parts of the plants are collected at certain times of the day, weak, month or year in order to obtain their full therapeutic effects. It is based upon their religious beliefs as well as their concept of time. To them day and night, month and season have got their specific importance for preparation and administration of medicine. Widows are not allowed to visit the medicine men while preparing or administering the drugs. They never collect plants for medicines in night because they believe that plants sleep in the night. The spiritual and magical aspects of this practice can not be ignored. It has its own significance in the treatment of diseases. Their beliefs and practices go side by side. Their habitation in inaccessible area, weak economic condition and their beliefs compel them to prefer indigenous method of treatment.[199]

It is difficult for a tribal man to undergo modern medical treatment which involves a lot of financial pressure. Only a limited per cent of Indian rural population has facilities for state managed health services. The condition of Odisha is still worse in the tribal pocket. So tribals in such a situation resort to indigenous physiotherapeutic method of treatment which is mainly based on plants. They are compelled to take traditional healing system because of its easy accessibility, low cost, cultural acceptability, elaborate patient-healer interaction, long term family association, friendly attitude of the medicinemen and many other socio-economic and religious causes.

Approximately 85 per cent of the rural population of India depends upon wild varieties of plants for the treatment of various diseases they suffer from. But urbanisation, rapid industrialisation and acculturation affected the tribal environment and culture. Due to destruction of forests, spread of harmful chemicals, introduction of alien species and over-exploitation of the natural resources a number of plants have already disappeared and others are awaiting the similar fate. It is therefore important to preserve the medicinal plants and empirical indigenous knowledge on plant resources before it is lost. It will be an option to cure the health hazards of the modern man whether tribal or non-tribal for all times to come.

References

1. J.C. Kurian, *Plants that Heal*, Oriental Watchman Publishing House, Pune, 1995, vii.
2. Malaya Kumar Mishra, *Udbhida Parichaya*, (Oriya), Berhampur University, 1998, 3.
3. S.K. Jain, *Medicinal Plants*, National Book Trust, New Delhi, 1968, 3.
4. N.K. Behura and K.K. Mohanty, *Tribal Orissa*, Dominant Publishers, New Delhi, 2006, 117-118.
5. *Adivasi*, Vol. XXXVII No. 2, December, 1997, Scheduled Castes and Scheduled Tribes Research and Training Institute, (herein after SCSTRTI), Bhubaneswar, 111-V.
6. G.N. Mohanty and A.K. Maharana, "The Santal Therapy Vis-a-Vis Animal Based Medicines", *Adivasi,* Vol. 46, No. 1, SCSTRTI, June, 2006, 1-2.
7. Personal Communication during fieldwork with Raghunath Mallik, (Medicine man), Upara Haridabadi, Chikiti, Ganjam, on 30.12.2010.
8. Sudipta Rath and P.K. Acharya, "Healing Pratices of Tribal Medicine Men in Mayurbhanj District of Orissa", *Adivasi*, Vol.-46, No. 1, SCSTRTI, Bhubaneswar, 11-12.
9. N. Patnaik, F. Bara and A. Mall, "Herbal Medicines of Dongrias", *Adivasi*, Vol. XXVI, No. 4, December, 1986, SCSTRTI, Bhubaneswar, 1-2.
10. Santosh Kumar Senapati, *Ethnobiological Studies on Mahendragiri Range of Hills of Eastern Ghats,* Orissa, Unpublished thesis, Berhampur University, 2005, 20.

11. N. Patnaik, *et al.*, *op. cit.*, 2.
12. Soumit Kumar Behera, Anima Panda, Susanta Ku. Behera and Malaya Kumar Misra "Medicinal Plants used by Kondha Tribe of Orissa." *Indian Journal of Traditional Knowledge*, Vol. V (4), October, 2006, 523-524.
13. Bijayalaxmi Dash and Nirmal Chandra Dash, *Kondhs: An Ethnobotanical Study*, Amadeus Press, 2009, 80.
14. *Ibid.*, 81.
15. Personal communication during the fieldwork with Surendra Mallick (Medicine man), Bhaliaguda, Kukudakhandi, Ganjam, on 29.12.2010.
16. N. Pattnaik, *et al.*, *op. cit.*, 2.
17. Soumit Kumar Behera, *et al.*, *op. cit.*., 523.
18. Bijayalaxmi Dash and Nirmal Chandra Dash, *op. cit.*, 78.
19. Personal communication during the fieldwork with Surendra Mallick, Bhaliaguda, Kukudakhandi, Ganjam, on 29.12.2010.
20. N. Patnaik, *et al.*, *op. cit.*, 2.
21. Bijayalaxmi Dash and Nirmal Chandra Dash, *op. cit.*, 164.
22. Soumit Kumar Behera, *et al.*, *op. cit.*, 526.
23. Bijayalaxmi Dash and Nirmal Chandra Dash, *op. cit.*, 64-88.
24. P.K. Dash and M. K. Mishra, "Some Medicinal Plants Among Kondhs Around Chandrapur (Koraput)", *Journal of Economic and Taxonomic Botany*, Vol. 12, No. 1, 1988, 107.
25. Sudhansu Sekhar Dash, Malaya Kumar Mishra, "Tribal Uses of Plants from Narayana Patna Region of Koraput District", Orissa, *Ancient Science of Life*, Vol. No. XV, January, 1996, 234-235.
26. *Ibid.*, 235.
27. N.K. Behura and K.K. Mohanti, *Tribal Orissa: Readings in Social Anthropology*, Dominant Publisher, New Delhi, 2006, 126.
28. Personal Communication during the fieldwork with Anirudha Dehuri (Medicine man), Jamijhori, Khajuripada, Kandhamal, on 24.05.2010.
29. Soumit Kumar Behera, *et al.*, *op. cit.*, 520-524.
30. Bijayalaxmi Dash and Nirmal Chandra Dash, *op. cit.*, 48-66.
31. *Ibid.*, 70-84.
32. Sudhansu Sekhar Dash and Malaya Kumar Mishra, *op. cit.*, 231-234.

33. P.K. Das and M.K. Mishra, "Some Medicinal Plants used by the Tribals of Deomali and Adjacent Areas of Koraput District, Orissa", *Indian Journal of Forestry*, Vol. 10 (4), 1987, 303.
34. Personal communication during the fieldwork with Anirudha Dehuri (Medicine man), Jamijhori, Khajuripada, Kandhamal, on 24.05.2010.
35. Sudhansu Sekhar Dash and Malaya Kumar Mishra, *op. cit.*, 233.
36. Personal communication during fieldwork with Bholanatha Pradhan (Medicine man), Gatamala, G. Udayagiri, Kandhamal, on 22.05.2010.
37. Soumit Kumar Behera, *et al.*, *op. cit.*, 520-526.
38. J.C. Kurian, *op. cit.*, 23.
39. Bijayalaxmi Dash and Nirmal Chandra Dash, *op. cit.*, 50.
40. *Ibid.*, 77.
41. N. Patnaik, *et al.*, *op. cit.*, 2.
42. Soumit Kumar Behera, *et al.*, *op. cit.*, 521-527.
43. Bijayalaxmi Dash and Nirmal Chandra Dash, *op. cit.*, 71-83.
44. *Ibid.*, 71-77.
45. *Ibid.*, 46-52.
46. *Ibid.*, 70-77.
47. Soumit Kumar Behera, *et al.*, 520-527.
48. Bijayalaxmi Dash and Nirmal Chandra Dash, *op. cit.*, 53-64.
49. Personal communication during the fieldwork with Raghunath Mallik (Medicine man), Upara Haridabadi, Chikiti, Ganjam, on 30. 12. 2010.
50. Bijayalaxmi Dash and Nirmal Chandra Dash, *op. cit.*, 53-68.
51. *Ibid.*, 70-75.
52. Sudhansu Sekhar Dash and Malaya Kumar Mishra, *op. cit.*, 232-234.
53. N. Patnaik, *et al.*, *op. cit.*, 3.
54. Soumit Kumar Behera, *et al.*, *op. cit.*, 521.
55. J.C. Kurian, *op. cit.*, 246.
56. Bijayalaxmi Dash and Nirmal Chandra Dash, *op. cit.*, 77.
57. N. Patnaik, et. al, *op. cit.*, 3.
58. Soumit Kumar Behera, *et al.*, *op. cit.*, 522-527.

59. Personal communication during the fieldwork with Durjyo Hikka (Medicine man), Rajanapanasaguda, Laxmipur, Koraput, on 10.06.2010.
60. S.K. Jain, *op. cit.*, 17.
61. Personal communication during the fieldwork with Saru Kilo (Medicine man), Disariguda, Khairiput, Malkangiri, on 12.06.2010.
62. Bijayalaxmi Dash and Nirmal Chandra Dash, *op. cit.*, 79-87.
63. *Ibid.*, 64-73.
64. J. C. Kurian, *op. cit.*, 21.
65. Soumit Kumar Behera, *et al.*, *op. cit.*, 524-527.
66. *Ibid.*, 520-521.
67. Personal communication during the fieldwork with Raibari Mallik *(Bejuni)*, Lunduriguda, Kukudakhandi, Ganjam on 29.12.2010.
68. Soumit Kumar Behera, *et al.*, *op. cit.*, 526-527.
69. Personal communication during fieldwork with Saru Kilo (Medicine man), Dasiriguda, Khairiput, Malkangiri on 12.06.2010.
70. Bijayalaxmi Dash and Nirmal Chandra Dash, *op. cit.*, 87.
71. S.K. Jain, *op. cit.*, 35.
72. N. Patnaik, *et al.*, *op. cit.*, 3.
73. Bijayalaxmi Dash and Nirmal Chandra Dash, *op. cit.*, 74-75.
74. N.K. Behura and K. K. Mohanti, *op. cit.*, 130.
75. J.C. Kurian, *op., cit.*, 20.
76. Bijayalaxmi Dash and Nirmal Chandra Dash, *op. cit.*, 75-76.
77. J.C. Kurian, *op. cit.*, 120.
78. N.K. Behura and K. K. Mohanti, *op. cit.*, 130.
79. Soumit Kumar Behera, *et al.*, *op. cit.*, 521-522.
80. Bijayalaxmi Dash and Nirmal Chandra Dash, *op. cit.*, 62.
81. *Ibid.*, 71-72.
82. Soumit Kumar Behera, *et al.*, *op. cit.*, 522-527.
83. Bijayalaxmi Dash and Nirmal Chandra Dash, *op. cit.*, 61.
84. N. Patnaik, *et al.*, *op. cit.*, 3.
85. Bijayalaxmi Dash and Nirmal Chandra Dash, *op. cit.*, 48-49.
86. *Ibid.*, 65-66.

87. Pramod Mishra, *op. cit.*, 183.
88. N. Patnaik, *et.al*, *op. cit.*, 3.
89. "Tribal Medicine and Medicinemen an Exploratory Study of the Didayi of Orissa", in *Adivasi*, Vol. XXXVII, No. 2, December, 1997, 101.
90. N. Patnaik, *et al.*, *op. cit.*, 3.
91. Soumit Kumar Behera, *et al.*, *op. cit.*, 521-522.
92. Bijayalaxmi Dash and Nirmal Chandra Dash, *op. cit.*, 78-79.
93. Sudhansu Sekhar Dash and Malaya Kumar Mishra, *op. cit.*, 233-234.
94. Personal communication during the fieldwork with Surendra Mallik (Medicine man), Bhaliaguda, Kukudakhandi, Ganjam on 29.12.2010.
95. Soumit Kumar Behera, *op. cit.*, 520-526.
96. Personal Communication during the fieldwork with Raibari Mallik, *Bejuni*, Lunduriguda, Kukudakhandi, Ganjam on 29.12.2010.
97. Bijayalaxmi Dash and Nirmal Chandra Dash, *op. cit.*, 58-60.
98. *Ibid.*, 74-77.
99. Personal communication during the fieldwork with Raibari Mallik, *Bejuni*, Lunduriguda, Kukudakhandi, Ganjam on 29.12.2010.
100. Sudhansu Sekhar Dash and Malaya Kumar Mishra, *op. cit.*, 233-234.
101. Personal communication during the fieldwork with Dandapani Knhor (Medicine man) Lambabadi, Khajuripada, Kandhamal, on 20.05.2010.
102. N. Patnaik, *et al.*, *op. cit.*, 3.
103. Soumit Kumar Behera *et al.*, *op. cit.*, 520-521.
104. Bijayalaxmi Dash and Nirmal Chandra Dash, *op. cit.*, 62.
105. "Tribal Medicine and Medicinemen an Exploratory Study of the Bondo of Orissa", in *Adivasi*, Vol. XXXVII, No. 2, December, SCSTRTI, Bhubaneswar, 1997, 64.
106. Bijayalaxmi Dash and Nirmal Chandra Dash, *op. cit.*, 75.
107. *Ibid.*, 84.
108. Sudhansu Sekhar Dash and Malay Kumar Mishra, *op .cit.*, 231.
109. N.K. Behura, K.K. Mohanti, *op. cit.*, 221-222.

110. J.C. Kurian, *op. cit.*, 26-27.

111. Soumit Kumar Behera, *et al.*, *op. cit.*, 522-524.

112. Bijayalaxmi Dash and Nirmal Chandra Dash, *op. cit.*, 65.

113. Soumit Kumar Behera, *et al.*, *op. cit.*, 522.

114. Personal Communication during the fieldwork with Dirjyo Hikka (Medicine man), Rajanapanasaguda, Laxmipur, Koraput, on 10.06.2010.

115. J.C. Kurian, *op. cit.*, 26.

116. Personal Communication during fieldwork with Surendra Mallik (Medicine man), Bhaliaguda, Kukudakhandi, Ganjam, on 29.12.2010.

117. N. Patnaik, *et al.*, *op. cit.*, 3.

118. *Ibid.*, 4.

119. Soumit Kumar Behera, *et al.*, *op. cit.*, 520-526.

120. N.K. Behura and K.K. Mohanti, *op. cit.*, 123.

121. G. Bulliyya, J.K. Naik and G. Mallik, "Indigenous Health Care Practices among the Kondh Tribal Communities of Orissa, India", in Awadesh N. Sharma, *et al.*, (eds.) *Indigenous Health Care and Ethnomedicine*, Sarup and Sons, New Delhi, 2006, 66.

122. Bijayalaxmi Dash and Nirmal Chandra Dash, *op. cit.*, 55-56.

123. Sudipta Rath, "Indigenous Tribal Healers and their Knowledge in Healthcare Practices," in Jyotsna Mohanty, (ed.), *Tribal Health, Culture and Development in Orissa*, Kamla Nehru Women's College, Bhubaneswar, 2004, 192.

124. G. Bulliyya, *et al.*, *op. cit.*, 65.

125. S.K. Jain, *op. cit.*, 35.

126. Sudhansu Sekhar Dash and Malaya Kumar Mishra, *op. cit.*, 232.

127. Soumit Kumar Behera, *et al.*, *op. cit.*, 522-523.

128. N. Patnaik, *et al.*, *op. cit.*, 4.

129. Soumit Kumar Behera, *et al.*, *op. cit.*, 520-526.

130. G. Bulliyya, *et al.*, *op. cit.*, 65.

131. Bijayalaxmi Dash and Nirmal Chandra Dash, *op. cit.*, 141.

132. G. Bulliyya, *et al.*, *op. cit.*, 67.

133. *The Kandha of Orissa*, SCSTRTI, Bhubaneswar, 2006, 212.

134. N. Patnaik, *et al.*, *op. cit.*, 4.

135. Personal Communication during fieldwork with Sahadev Dehuri, (Medicine man), Jamujhari, Khajuripada, Kandhamala, on 24.05.2010.
136. Bijayalaxmi Dash and Nirmal Chandra Dash, *op. cit.*, 65-71.
137. G. Bulliyya, *et al.*, *op. cit.*, 65.
138. "Tribal Medicine and Medicinemen an Exploratory Study of the Didayi of Orissa", in *Adivasi*, Vol. XXXVI, No. 2, December, SCSTRTI, Bhubaneswar, 1997, 99.
139. P.K. Dash and M.K. Mishra, *op. cit.*, 107.
140. N. Pattnaik. *et al.*, *op. cit.*, 4.
141. Personal Communication during fieldwork with Sahadev Dehuri (Medicine man) Jamujhari, Khajuripada, Kandhamal on 24.05.2010.
142. Bijayalaxmi Dash and Nirmal Chandra Dash, *op. cit.*, 59-60.
143. N. Patnaik, *et al.*, *op. cit.*, 4.
144. "Tribal Medicine and Medicinemen an Exploratory Study of the Bondo of Orissa", in *Adivasi*, Vol XXXVII, No. 2, December, SCSTRTI, Bhubaneswar, 1997, 68.
145. N.K. Behura *et al.*, *op. cit.*, 131.
146. Sudhansu Sekhar Dash and Malay Kumar Mishra, *op. cit.*, 232.
147. Soumit Kumar Behera, *et al.*, *op. cit.*, 521-524.
148. Sudipta Rath, *op. cit.*, 194.
149. Promod Misra, *op. cit.*, 181.
150. Personal Communication during fieldwork with Baada Malik, Rebringia, Baliguda, Kandhamal, on 23.05.2010.
151. J.C. Kurian, *op. cit.*, 313.
152. *Ibid.*, 154.
153. *Ibid.*, 113.
154. Soumit Kumar Behera, *et al.*, *op. cit.*, 522.
155. Personal Communication during fieldwork with Raibari Mallik *Bejuni*, Lunduriguda, Kukudakhandi, Ganjam, on 29.12.2010.
156. Personal Communication during fieldwork with Surendra Mallik, (Medicine man), Bhalliaguda, Kukudakhandi, Ganjam on 29.12.2010.
157. Bijayalaxmi Dash and Nirmal Chandra Dash, *op. cit.*, 78-79.
158. *Ibid.*, 65.

159. Personal Communication during fieldwork with Dirjyo Hikka, (Medicine man) Rajanapanasaguda, Laxmipur, Koraput, on 10.06.2010 .
160. Pramod Misra, *op. cit.*, 179-180.
161. Bijayalaxmi Dash and Nirmal Chandra Dash, *op. cit.*, 64-65.
162. J.C. Kurian, *op. cit.*, 30.
163. N. Patnaik, *et al.*, *op. cit.*, 4.
164. Bijayalaxmi Dash and Nirmal Chandra Dash, *op. cit.*, 45-57.
165. *Ibid.*, 63-64.
166. "Tribal Medicine and Medicinemen an Exploratory Study of the Bondo of Orissa", in *Adivasi*, Vol. XXXVII, No. 2, December, 1997, SCSTRTI, Bhubaneswar, 65-68.
167. Personal Communication during fieldwork with Surendra Mallik, Bhaliaguda, Kukudakhandi, Ganjam on 29.12.2010.
168. Personal Communication during fieldwork with Raibari Mallik, *Bejuni*, Lunduriguda, Kukudakhandi, Ganjam on 29.12.2010.
169. Sudipta Rath, *op. cit.*, 191.
170. G. Bulliyya, *et.al.*, *op. cit.*, 68.
171. N.K. Behura *et al.*, *op. cit.*, 128.
172. Soumit Kumar Behera, *et al.*, *op. cit.*, 520.
173. Personal Communication during fieldwork with Raghunath Mallik (Medicine man), Upara Haridabadi, Chikiti, Ganjam on 30.12.2010.
174. N. Patnaik. *et al.*, *op. cit.*, 4.
175. Personal Communication during field work with Raghunath Mallik, (Medicine man), Upara Haridabadi, Chikiti, Ganjam on 30.12.2010.
176. Bijayalaxmi Dash and Nirmal Chandra Dash, *op. cit.*, 50-56.
177. J.C. Kurian, *op., cit.*, 61.
178. "Tribal Medicine and Medicinemen an Exploratory Study of the Didayi of Orissa", in *Adivasi*, Vol. XXXVII, No.2, , December 1997, SCSTRTI, Bhubaneswar, 97.
179. Bijayalaxmi Dash and Nirmal Chandra Dash, *op. cit.*, 136-140.
180. *Ibid.*, 58.
181. J.C. Kurian, *op. cit.*, 21-31.
182. Personal Communication during fieldwork with Surendra Mallik (Medicine man), Bhaliaguda, Kukudakhandi, Ganjam, on 29.12.2010.

183. J.C. Kurian, *op. cit.*, 297.
184. Promod Misra, *op. cit.*, 186.
185. Soumit Kumar Behera, *et al.*, *op. cit.*, 522.
186. Personal Communication during field work with Sahadev Dehuri (Medicine man), Jamujhari, Khajuripada, Kandhamal on 24.05.2010.
187. Bijayalaxmi Dash and Nirmal Chandra Dash, *op. cit.*, 69-71.
188. Personal Communication during fieldwork with Taru Pradhan, (Medicine man), Jharijhula, Chakapad, Kandhamal on 25.05.2010.
189. Soumit Kumar Behera, *et al.*, *op. cit.*, 526.
190. S.K. Jain, *op. cit.*, 34-35.
191. P.K. Das and M.K. Mishra, *op. cit.*, 105.
192. J.C. Kurian, *op. cit.*, 313.
193. *Ibid.*, 273.
194. Personal Communication during fieldwork with Taru Pradhan, (Medicine man), Jharijhula, Chakapad, Kandhamal, on 25.05.2010.
195. Bijayalaxmi Dash and Nirmal Chandra Dash, *op. cit.*, 113.
196. J.C. Kurian, *op. cit.*, 49.
197. Personal Communication during fieldwork with Surendra Mallik, (Medicine man), Bhaliaguda, Kukudakhandi, Ganjam, on 29.12.2010.
198. Bijayalaxmi Dash and Nirmal Chandra Dash, *op. cit.*, 118.
199. Personal Communication during the field work, with Surendra Mallick (Medicine man), Bhaliaguda, Kukudakhandi Ganjam on 29.12.2010.

5

Tribal Medicine *versus* Modern Medicine

A study of medical systems and health is very interesting in the Indian context because this country possesses an immense heterogeneity in medical beliefs and practices. In addition to the well known and wide spread medical systems such as Ayurveda, Allopathy, Unani and Homoeopathy, there are various types of localised folk and tribal medical beliefs and practices often based on magic and sorcery. Since five decades or so there is no dearth of medical anthropological research in India. These studies mainly have focused their attention on both tribal and less developed rural communities. Besides a description of their beliefs and practices about illness and medicine, the interaction between modern and traditional medical systems also forms an important aspect of this study.[1]

Since time immemorial, diseases have been a part of human life and they sometimes have threatened the existence of human race. Consequently, man has invented a host of devices through a trial and error method to control the vagaries of various diseases. The concepts of aetiology of illness, methods of diagnosis and treatment with ideas of prophylaxis have been developed and preserved as the traditional lore of every society. Most of this knowledge has been acquired by men not intentionally, but through their experiences in everyday life. As a result, they have evolved a body of practical, common sense knowledge. The basic character of this knowledge and the common feature expressed by the methods and techniques developed by them are that they are symbolic and expressive rather than scientific and experimental.[2]

Every human society in the world, irrespective of its degree of cultural and material simplicity or complexity has maintained an effective medical system and possessed empirically tested knowledge about aetiology and curing to cope with the diseases which threaten the well-being of its members.[3] Very often, these traditional medical beliefs and practices may not appear quite rational when viewed from the conceptual framework of modern scientific medicine. But it worked satisfactorily with the people who made use of it.

Preservation of health is a duty. Good health is a vital part of the great experience of living. Every age has made new discoveries and inventions about health, thereby providing man with new weapons to fight disease. Health is a matter which affects not only each one of us as individuals but also the community in which we live. Human body is regarded as the most important means to attain highest physical and spiritual goals in life. One must look after one's physical body first leaving other worldly things aside because in the absence of body, nothing will have existence.[4]

The concept of health, disease, treatment, life and death among the tribes is as varied as their culture. Sick people as cultural beings have over time developed social institutions, aetiological theories and therapeutic techniques in order to enable them to cope with the social and other dislocations occasioned by illness induced disability. All cultures have a set of ideas for defining and treating disease, ways of prescribing cures. Human society has created an adoptive strategy to counter disease.[5] People very often use more than one medicine for the treatment of an ailment. The medicine varies according to the symptoms as well as secondary effects. Again depending on the availability sometimes alternative plants are used for more than one disease. Tribal people categorise the disease into two parts – (i) related to body, i.e., physiological and (ii) related to mind and divine powers, i.e., psychosomatic. The bodily ailments are treated by using herbal medicines coupled with animal parts/products and minerals whereas the other is treated through magico-religious means.[6]

The success of a medical system can be evaluated by examining how the people utilise this knowledge to maintain their health and living in harmony with their environment. While going through the evolutionary history of mankind, one can find that the notion of health, disease and healing practices constitute an important part of the human culture itself. Diseases threatened man's existence on earth and human societies were forced to invent a pharmacopoeia and to develop therapeutic measures to win over the challenges met from the environment.

General health status of the tribals is poor as compared to the modern society. They suffer from some distinct health problems not because they have some specific type of health but because of specific placement in unhygienic areas and environment in which they live. Because of widely varying geo-climatic and ecological conditions and the different tribal societies have some specific health issues and problems of their own. The health status of the tribals is affected by the factors like widespread poverty, illiteracy, malnutrition, non availability of safe drinking water and insanitary living condition. A tribal in general, hardly makes distinction in the magnitude of the disease. They have a definite means for identifying and classifying various diseases.[7]

The Kondhs do primarily depend upon forest for their livelihood. The state with semi evergreen and deciduous vegetation is endowed with various wild plants and natural resources. Due to their constant association with forest for meeting their everyday requirements, they have developed a very good knowledge about the use of wild plants in various aspects of their life. They solely depend upon forest for their entire medicine.[8] It is noticeable that the Kondhs who are living in a hostile environment can manage to lead an active life with the help of their own medical practices and cultural etiquette. Their religious beliefs, cultural values and customs help them to regulate their activities and to exploit the resources of their environment without tilting its ecological balance.

Oxford dictionary defines "medicine" as an art of restoring and preserving health. The institution of medicine is as old as mankind. It has been a part and parcel of human society since the evolution of disease.[9] The foundation of human life and other forms of life on earth is varied and ample. Human beings transform the natural order of their habitat into a moral order or natural ecology to cultural ecology by means of culture. Tribal societies throughout the world have respective system of medicine for primary health needs.[10]

Health has been regulated in traditional communities by the medicine man or shaman on the basis of sound ecological factors, although neither the medicine man nor the patient may have been consciously aware of the underlying basis of treatment. The medicine man derives all his medicines from the nature, which includes plant parts, animal matter and minerals. As medicines are the products from the forest, there is no degenerating effect. All the medicines are available in environment to which the tribal community has adopted themselves. They do not consider any disease as the cause of neglect of body or its organs. They consider disease as an integral part of the life process. They believe that disease means unhappiness, fear, tragedy and suffering. They accept displeasure of supernatural entities as the cause of disease and sickness.[11]

Ethno-medicine is still persisting in the Kondh communities even after introduction of modern medicine since a number of decades. Since time immemorial, they have been using plant resources for various purposes. Human beings are dependent on plants either directly or indirectly. Of course, its former popularity and reliability has considerably eroded and a number of tribal's are now exploiting the facilities of modern medicine in addition to ethno-medicine.

Medicine man play a vital role in Kondh community. Their own community recognises them as competent to provide health care by using various herbal medicines. In thousands of Kondh dominated villages where hardly any medical facilities exist, they are the only source of support and hope for survival. It is believed that the knowledge of herbal medicine has been received from god in dream and this knowledge is orally transmitted from generation to generation.[12] The knowledge of these medicines is confined to the medicine man alone. He does not disclose this knowledge for fear that by doing so he may lose his powers of healing. Certain plants species like *kara mara, bidi mara, raga mara* and *bichu mara* for medicine can only be found under the guidance of the gods. The *kutaka's* divine powers enable the healer to locate these species but if he attempts to use them as medicines without the god's instruction, the plants will lose their efficacy. A traditional medical system is a collection of experiences and knowledge relating to the diagnosis of an illness, and its cure.[13] The use of traditional medicine still prevails among Kondhs although the modern medicine is now available free of charge.

However, by a close observation one can find out that traditional ethno-medicine is still viable and it plays a commendable role in the treatment of ailments. Modern medicine though has a primarily biological orientation, factors of health, sickness, aetiology of disease and their indigenous methods of treatment are all deeply rooted in the cultural history of the people. Disease and suffering are the normal events of life. In tribal societies which are still anchored in the domain of traditionalism, one's first option is ethnic healing methods and advice of ethnic healers because modern methods of treatment have not yet come handy for tribals.[14]

There are various favourable factors responsible for the survival of indigenous method of treatment. The majority of curative centres like hospitals, dispensaries, etc., are located in urban areas. So the people seeking medical assistance have to travel long distance to reach the nearest hospital. The tribals often do not have either the resources or the ability to go to the hospitals in the urban areas. So they look forward to ethno-medicine which is easily available in their own locality for protecting them from the ailments.

People have to spend a lot of money for getting efficient treatment from the private hospitals. Only cheap medicines are available from the government hospitals. For most of the costly medicines, the doctors are used to give prescription notes and the patients have to buy them from the medical stores outside the hospital. Most of the Kondh people cannot afford this treatment. So they depend upon ethno-medicine which is available free of cost from the medicine man.

Ethno-medicine is very effective in checking a number of diseases. The magico-religious therapy of Disari and Jani is aided by the powerful tool of suggestions, which is very helpful in bringing about cure. The rituals of shamans have much psychological impact upon the patients and he believes that the efficient techniques of shaman can remove his illness.[15]

The plant, animal and mineral matters used in the drug therapy of ethno-medicine have real physiotherapeutic effect upon the patients. The Kondhs have a rich knowledge about the medicinal properties of various plants and they use them effectively in the treatment of diseases. In addition to this, they have other techniques like diet control, fasting, massage, bone-setting, etc., to face various types of ailments.

Most of the Kondhs have faith that ethno-medicine is harmless and more suitable for the body vis-à-vis modern medicine. As plants, minerals and animal materials obtained from nature are used for the preparation of medicine, its function inside the body is assumed to be quite natural and rejuvenating. They hold the belief that even though modern medicine gives quick relief, it is harmful to the body. After healing one's illness, the harmful principles of the medicine can cause another disease in the same person sometime later.

It is found that when both ethno and modern medicines are available, the patients or their relatives take some arbitrary decisions about what kind of medicine is suitable for the treatment of a particular disease. Often they approach the medicine man for minor ailments and go to a hospital for serious diseases. In some cases, the medicine man used to carry out a second screening. After examining the patient, he refers the more complicated cases to a hospital.

As a result of screening, modern medicines get the more complicated and serious cases while ethno-medicines get only cases of minor illness. So, the percentage of success is higher in case of ethno-medicine than in case of modern medicine. Thus the screening is favourable to the ethno-medicine and contributes to its apparent efficiency.[16]

The practitioner of ethno-medicine is an insider to the community and the patients have personal relationships with him. The medicine man is related to the patient as a friend, kinsman, etc. So their relationship is very cordial and informal. After diagnosis, the medicine man explains to the patient the causes and remedies of the illness. Thus along with the healer, the patient also has an active role in the treatment procedure. This ensures full co-operation of the patient with the healer and their joint effort brings success easily. From a medicine man or witchdoctor a tribal patient does not merely receive a physical health treatment but something much more than that. He gets moral support which he cannot get from modern doctor.[17]

The relationship between a patient and a doctor is formal and they are representatives of two different cultures. The doctor asks a number of questions to the patient about the disease and seldom explains the cause and remedy of the illness. The interest of the doctor in the patient is limited to the disease, its diagnosis and treatment. Lack of respect for indigenous culture and inattention towards the patient are sometimes responsible for the non-acceptance and distrust of the tribal people towards modern medicine. A medical practice having its roots in alien culture has chances of conflict between different cultural values.[18] One of the greatest strength of tribal systems of medicine is the involvement of group in therapy. The role and responsibilities of kin, lineage-mates and villagers who form the therapy management group in health seeking and helping in therapeutic outcomes is a remarkable property of this system.

However ethno-medicine of the Kondhs is now influenced by a number of forces external to the community, which are capable of bringing out changes in this traditional system. As a part of the tribal welfare programmes, the government has opened a number of curative centres like hospitals, dispensaries and Primary Health Centres (PHC) in the tribal area and also has employed mobile dispensaries to improve the availability of medical facilities for them. In addition to this, modern medicine is also available to them from a number of private nursing homes and hospitals, functioning in rural areas within an easily reachable distance from the abode of the tribal's. However on many occasions, the Kondh people show much reluctance in accepting modern medicine for the treatment of diseases. It is observed that sometime their resistance towards modern medicine is disease specific. They accept modern medicine for certain diseases but reject it for some others. This selective approach is a major hurdle for the health personnel in the successful implementation of their programmes.[19]

The treatment of diseases among the tribes may not be reasonable but it will be wrong to assume that it has no science. It rather moves in a way, which covers not only a scientific principle but also involves the society at large to overcome the catastrophe. The primitives have some scientific knowledge which they gather/learn through experience. The traditional people have learnt through trial and error method. But this method does not exist in isolation, rather is a part of their entire socio-cultural, religious system. Their own system of health is an integral part of their culture. They have used wild plants and herbs over centuries to fight against disease and as sources of food and energy. They have medicines for maladies ranging from cardiac disorder to dog-bite. They use castor seeds as contraceptive. If their knowledge is acknowledged and recorded properly, it can open up new vista of various antidotes against many diseases.

The study of the medical systems of Kondh society needs urgent attention, considering the influence of various agents which are inducing rapid changes in this section of the population. Most of the Kondhs are no longer enjoying complete isolation from other human groups and rapid social changes can be noticed due to the contact with the people of other cultures. The various welfare measures of the government to raise the standard of life of the tribals have accelerated the pace of these changes. Now, a number of tribes are following the life-style of the non-tribal societies and their traditional norms, values, social institutions and subsistence pattern have undergone vital transformation. So steps must be taken to study the ethno medical practices of the tribals and to record all the efficacious medicines used by them, before they are lost. Modern medicine has lot of side effects. It is expensive and beyond the reach of lay man. But ethno medicine is less toxic, effective and within the reach of lay man, besides being less expensive. As the modern medicine is having different adverse results and alarming adverse side effects, we need to remember that the mother of all indigenous medicines is the tribal medicine practiced by the communities living in close harmony with the eco-system. Thus its documentation is an urgent need and it should be translated in all the available traditional knowledge as per international standards and safeguard the patenting rights of the stake holders. It has to be done in relatively more details with respect to the information like symptoms, methods of indigenous preparation, sources of information, modes of administration and the final outcome of the treatment.[20] Hence, it is wise to train the traditional medicine man scientifically who can be utilised for the benefit of the community. They can provide the service when the tribals are in need. The traditional system does not come in conflict with the modern system of medicine as both are seen to co-exist. As the traditional medicine man have great influence over the people, their service should be utilised as the health educators of the community.

With the large-scale immigration of non tribals from the plains, a lot of changes have occurred among the tribes. The land-hungry and hard working non-tribals have converted large areas of forests into agricultural fields and plantations. They have introduced the cultivation of various cash crops like rubber, pepper, tea, cardamom, lemongrass, ginger etc. Often they have grabbed the land of the tribals and driven them to the interior areas of forests. This change of habitat adversely affected the life of the Kondh people. After large-scale deforestation they could not get the traditional items of food from the forest. They are confronted with the scarcity of medicinal plants and animal matter also. For the first time in their history they are getting exposed to the vices of adulteration and pollution with the march of time. After the contact with non-tribal's and also due to the change in consumption pattern, new diseases came into existence among them. Most of these diseases were formerly unknown.[21] So the tribal medicine man find it difficult to treat these new diseases. At this juncture, modern medicine has played a crucial role. When they found that their ethno-medicine was ineffective in curing the new diseases, some of them sought the assistance of modern medicine. From their experience, they have realised that modern medicine is very efficient in healing the new ailments. However, even after they have started using modern medicine, ethno-medicine has continued to play a significant role in their health care. They have been using both systems of medicine according to the nature of disease aetiology.

In fact, the ethno-medicine of tribals is in a process of change due to the interaction with other cultures. Initially, the non-tribal immigrants from the plains influenced the tribal culture in a big way. Their own system of health care is being replaced by the state sponsored hospitals, primary health centres, community health centres and private dispensaries. The situation of traditional tribal medicine is rapidly changing as the government sponsored modern allopathic medicine is wiping out the traditional medicine from tribal areas.[22] Afterwards, the introduction of modern medicine into the tribal universe by both government and private agencies affected ethno-medicine and brought changes into this system. The knowledge system pertaining to health care and ethno-medicine is a part of traditional lore of the community and is always passed down from generation to generation through work processes and lore.[23] They follow the age-old medicinal combinations and healing techniques which they have inherited from their forefathers. This medical system is a closed one and it is neither experimental nor does it imbibe any knowledge from other cultures in any systematic way.

Ethno-medicine often cannot cope with the fast changes occurring in the community. Changes occurred in the habitat, subsistence pattern and dietary habits of the tribals and the close association with non-tribals tilted the balance of their traditional life. Along with these changes, acculturation brought forth many new diseases to them. Most of these diseases were not present among them in the past and hence the tribal medicine men are helpless to tackle them. It is quite natural that there is no medicine for maladies like pollution and adulteration in nature. The medicine men are not able to diagnose these causes which are not familiar to them. Although the traditional medicine has its own importance, the modern medicine plays a vital role. Tribals cannot diagnose the cause of the disease unless they have the knowledge of modern medical science.

They have a peculiar concept of fever and pain. Whenever a person feels pain in belly or suffers from fever suddenly and behaves abnormally, it is suspected that he has been attacked by an evil spirit. Evil spirit acts through a medium. It is also acknowledged by the society that few of them bear evil spirits.[24] They hardly make any difference between simple fever, malarial fever, pneumonia fever, typhoid fever, influenza etc. Similarly, the medicine man treats all stomach pains on the same footing whether it is dysenteric pain or constipation or some other intestinal disorder. So far as diagnosis of the disease is concerned, the tribals face great difficulty, particularly with anything different from the common disease of everyday occurrence. Most of the diseases are symptomatic.[25]

The medicine men of present age are not as competent as their predecessors. As the Kondhs in the past solely depended upon the forest for their food and medicine, the medicine men of those ages had a vast knowledge of the medicinal properties of flora and fauna. With the death of the old medicine men, considerable amount of knowledge was lost to the community. There are also some professional hindrances from a medicine man to his disciples. It is a commonly accepted notion that no teacher must teach all his techniques to his disciples. So the teachers used to hold back some of the important techniques from the disciples in order to keep up his supremacy. Some of the teachers want to reveal this knowledge in their last days. But very often they do not get any opportunity to do so and the precious medical knowledge is lost forever.

Forest happens to be the main sources of getting medicinal plants and animals. Large-scale deforestation and different laws restricting the use and exploitation of forest resources are adversely affecting the health and treatment in tribal society. A number of medicinal plants have been destroyed by the ruthless denudation of forest and today the medicine men suffer from the scarcity of these plants.[26] As the Kondhs do not have the habit of growing medicinal plants for their needs, they are always dependent upon natural sources. When these natural sources are destroyed they find it difficult to collect the various essential ingredients for medicinal preparations. This is equally applicable in the case of animal matter as ingredients of medicines. Deforestation also affects their availability.

The expertise of Kondh medicine man in the art of surgery is very crude and not sufficient for the successful treatment of complicated cases. Even though they have a good knowledge in the bone setting technique, they often commit mistakes when fractures are involved. Due to the mistakes in the treatment, some of the patients are found handicapped.

The sceptical attitude of the patients is a new problem confronting the practitioners of ethno-medicine. After getting little education and experiencing the capacity of modern medicine to impart speedy relief, the tribals, especially the youngsters, are more sceptical towards the efficacy of ethno-medical practices. This disbelief often retards the pace of the healing process. When the cure becomes very slow, the patients go to a hospital for availing the facilities of modern medicine for a speedy relief.[27]

Now-a-days some of the Kondh people are using ethno-medicine as a stopgap arrangement. When they cannot easily get modern medicine they depend upon ethno-medicine as the only medical facility available on the spot. But afterwards, they are used to go to the modern curative centres for further treatment. To cite an example, when somebody gets sick in the night or when he is inside the dense forest, there is no question of getting modern medicine immediately. So he quickly resorts to ethno-medicine which is available easily. If the illness persists, he goes to a hospital on the next day or when he comes out of the forest. So, such people have more belief in the quick relief brought by modern medicine and use ethno-medicine only as a stopgap arrangement.

After the advent of modern medicine, the Kondhs living in the border areas of forests used to take arbitrary decisions, based on their previous experiences, about what kind of disease is to be taken to which type of practitioners for treatment. Generally they show preference for the modern curative centres when afflicted by serious ailments and are satisfied with ethno-medicine for the treatment of minor illnesses and also maladies originating due to assumed supernatural causes. They have reduced the use of ethno-medicine for the treatment of even minor illnesses as a result of which it has lost its importance. However, the Kondhs living in dense forests do not take such arbitrary decisions and are availing the facilities of ethno-medicine for all their ailments.

The introduction of modern medicine has multiple impacts on the community in general and ethno-medical system in particular. This is a new system of medicine and all its methods and concepts of aetiology are alien to them. In the initial stage of its introduction, nobody bothered to avail its facilities, as people thought that it was not ideal for their culture and was not able to treat their illness. So this phase was a period of non contact between the tribal community and modern medicine. In this phase they continued the use of ethno-medicine for the treatment of various types of diseases. Because of the non-acceptance of the tribals, modern medicine could not do anything worthwhile for the health care of the Kondhs in its initial period of existence in the tribal areas.[28] Before going to any practitioner of modern medicine, Kondhs used to consult a medicine man of the community for any ailment. They are unwilling to spend money on modern medicine whereas they spend more money on the performance of customary death rituals. This is because of their strong faith on their tradition.

However, with the passage of time the Kondh people started availing the facilities of modern medicine. The efforts of the medical personnel, spread of education, increased mobility, close association with non-tribal immigrants, etc., influenced the way of thinking of the tribals and helped them to use modern medicine. Initially, the use of modern medicine by a small percentage of the people evoked a rebellious attitude among the rest of the community. Often the elders and medicine men ridiculed the people who used modern medicine which in their opinion is useless.

But the people who used modern medicine found its efficacy and capable of bringing speedy relief. Their favourable experience attracted others also who were sceptical to it earlier. So in course of time, more people started using this new system of therapy. Actually these people were ignorant of the underlying principles of modern medicine and of the ideas behind its mode of treatment. They are simply attracted by the curative ability of modern medicine.

Even in this phase of transition, Kondh people believe in supernatural causes for certain diseases. Magico-religious performances occupy a prominent place in the treatment of diseases. They believe that some diseases originate from the supernatural reasons like evil eye, sorcery, breach of taboo, anger of ancestral spirits and wrath of god. For the treatment of such diseases, they are still depending upon ethno-medicine and call their own magician instead of consulting a modern allopathic doctor. They strongly feel that doctors are quite helpless against such evil forces which can only be counteracted by the magical performances of the magicians.[29] While for certain other illnesses like chicken pox, measles and cholera they do not take any medicine at all because of certain beliefs. Religious performances occupy a prominent place in the treatment of such types of diseases.[30] Even if some modern medical help is resorted to, they are not of much help in curing these diseases. So the modern medical practitioner finds it difficult to eradicate the superstition that these are due to the wrath of god or goddess.

After prolonged experience with modern medicine the tribal's have realised that there is no miracle attached to its treatment and that it is not capable of healing every illness with equal effectiveness. They have also found that for the cure of certain illnesses, their own ethno-medicine is more efficient than the modern medicine. So gradually they have started selecting the type of medicine according to the nature of the illness. Without blindly following certain mode of treatment, they utilised the abilities of that medical treatment which is found efficacious for a particular illness. They have considered their own previous experiences while selecting one mode of medical treatment.

In the present age, one may be tempted to presume that modern medicine has taken over ethno-medicine and is the sole agent of health care for the Kondhs. But such an assumption would be far from the reality. The acceptance of modern medicine does not mean that people have lost all their faith in the ethno-medical system. Rather they choose different types of medicines for various illnesses according to the advantages of each one of them. So the old practices exist along with the new innovations. The acceptance of modern medicine does not mean that traditional ideas of disease aetiology have been superseded or that the cultural ramifications of specific illness have disappeared.[31]

The government at present is implementing a number of health programmes for the community; however it is observed that such programmes are not often successful in improving their standard of health. The medical practitioners and public health workers very often report that these tribal people do not utilise the medical, preventive and family planning facilities available to them. This is an important problem for the health planners and medical practitioners. The solution to this problem can be resolved only through a systematic study of the tribal concepts of aetiology, treatment of diseases and the role of a physician in the curing procedure. This can be proved by a systematic study on tribal medicine because the traditional approach establishes faith and assurance in the patients while the modern medicine lacks this.[32] Unless and until the reasons of failure are brought to light, the very health care programmes for the tribals cannot be successful.

Kondhs distinguish between physical and psychological diseases. The physical diseases include dermatitis, accidental injuries, pathogenic illness, fever, diarrhoea, leprosy and other physical ailments that results from food and exposure to the environment. The psychological illness include fear, anxiety, epilepsy, hysteria, chest pain, successive abortion, insanity, etc. said to be caused chiefly by evil spirits, supernatural powers and witchcraft. Tribals have much reluctance to accept modern medicine for the treatment of such supernatural diseases as they believe that no material medicine is efficacious in checking them. On the other hand, they resort to invoke the assistance of supernatural forces on such occasions.[33] While implementing the health programmes, proper consideration of such cultural inhibitions is necessary to avoid friction and misunderstanding between the tribals and the practitioners of modern medicine.

Kondh people take modern medicine only when the illness is an imported one or one which cannot be explained in terms of tribal logic. Of course in the last stage of diseases, when their magico-religious treatment fails, they go for modern treatment.[34] It is understood that the tribals possess effective methods in their ethno-medicine to treat those diseases which are present among them since remote past. However they do not know how to heal the newly imported diseases and therefore seek the assistance of modern medicine.

The policy of government to uplift the health condition of Kondhs through the introduction of modern medicine has a number of good as well as bad impacts on them. Many of them first rejected this new system of medicine. But with the passage of time, they have slowly started accepting it for the treatment of certain diseases. But the modern medicine often could not satisfy all their needs. So most of the people are now using the more efficacious elements of both the systems of medicine. The diseases originating from supernatural causes, as they believe are always treated by the traditional medicine man. Economic constraints and the isolation very often deter the people from using modern medicine. The results obtained from the household health survey show that ethno-medicine has a definite edge on modern medicine. Among those who are more tradition-oriented, this difference is clearer. While a good percentage of people shows no preference to any system of medicine.

Economic constraints form a major hurdle in availing the benefits of modern medicine. During the lean period, people struggle to purchase essential commodities. When somebody gets sick in this period, they depend upon ethno-medicine for cure. The patient may survive if the treatment is successful, otherwise he may die. The summer season is a vulnerable period and several epidemics break out during this time. Without getting proper care and effective medicine many people die. Scarcity of drinking water, unhygienic surrounding, hostile climate and inability to go for modern medicine increase the death rate.[35]

The non-availability of modern medicine is one of the major factors responsible for the continuous use of ethno-medicine. The Kondh's living in the remote areas have to walk 20 to 30 kilometers to reach a hospital. It is very difficult to bring a sick person from a remote village to the hospital as there are no communication facilities or convenient conveyance. Sometimes they bring the sick people by carrying in a wooden stretcher. So they are not getting proper medical treatment at right time.[36] Therefore when somebody is sick in such interior areas, he approaches the shaman or medicine man of the hamlet and follow his treatment.

In some cases, there is combined use of both modern and ethno-medicine. When a patient is very weak and unable to go to hospital by foot, he is used to take ethno-medicine from the medicine man of the hamlet. After a few days of treatment, there may be some relief in his condition and he may be able to move around without difficulty. Then he goes to a hospital in the nearby town and undergoes treatment there for getting a complete and speedy cure. Thus people select the type of medicine according to their need and pressure of circumstances.

In tribal areas, getting pure water is an acute problem. Generally the tribal people use stream or pond water during summer and rainy season. The stream and pond water is very dirty and polluted. This polluted water causes water-borne diseases like dysentery, diarrhoea, cholera, jaundice, etc.[37] Usually, the outside world comes to know about the onset of these epidemics very late as most of the tribal hamlets are situated inside dense forests in remote places. When news come in media, the concerned government departments suddenly become active and medical teams consisting of doctors, nurses and pharmacists are sent to the tribal hamlets for distributing medicine to the needy patients. But by the time the medical teams reach the hamlets, a number of patients are found to have passed away.

Moreover the response of the Kondhs towards medical teams is often negative. They believe that epidemics like measles and cholera originate by some supernatural causes. So no medicine is effective in checking them. They believe that use of medicine aggravates the anger of god and consequently the patient is likely to be serious. To avoid this unpleasant development, they say the medical personnel that nobody is sick in their house and they do not need any medical help. The Kondh women and children are very shy to face outsiders and often they run away when the medical team approaches a hamlet. Very often, it is found that they simply waste the medicines supplied to them by keeping them somewhere in the house.

So only through much persuasion, the Kondhs come forward to get themselves examined by the doctor and to receive the medicine. But the treatment of disease is sometimes ineffective because there is no way to know whether they will consume the medicine provided to them or not. With a short visit the medical personnel cannot enlighten them about the efficacy of modern medicine. So the effort to thrust upon modern medicine within a short time span makes them suspicious and they react towards it in a negative manner.[38]

The visit of medical teams during the outbreak of epidemics has a number of handicaps. The absence of rapport between the doctors and the tribals is a hindrance in giving modern medicine to them. The doctor is a strange person for them and the tribals by their very nature do not trust strangers. The medical personnel are also discouraged by the non-cooperative attitude of the tribals.

The most important drawback is that there are no follow-up visits or treatment after the visit. So the patients do not get medicine and care till their illness is completely cured. If a person who takes medicine from the medical team cannot get any relief because of the lack of availability of a full course of medicine, he is discouraged to take it again in future.

The communication between the doctor and the patient is often not satisfactory. The patient sometimes fails to convey the details of the symptoms properly or gives overemphasis to any one of them. Some of the patients may not be able to understand the method of medication ordered by the doctor. Often the doctors consider the tribals as ignorant people having a number of superstitions and do not attach the required seriousness to their disease. It is found that the patients always like the doctors who have some knowledge in their concepts of aetiology and treatment. They claim that some of the doctors have told them that for the cure of certain diseases the blessing of god is necessary.[39]

But some of the doctors are very busy and they do not ask any personal questions to their patients. His inquiry is limited to the disease only. People do not have much enthusiasm to follow the directions of such doctors. Often the doctors in the government hospitals belong to this category. The doctors of private hospitals spend more time with each patient and try to become friendly to him by asking many personal questions, which may not be often relevant for the treatment of illness. The tribals have much appreciation about this type of doctors and they contact them again when affected by a disease. Some of the doctors in the private hospitals may even give some concessions in the cost of treatment or allow the tribals to pay the money in convenient installments.

After contacting a doctor and receiving medicines from him, there are many other factors which become hindrance in the successful completion of the treatment. Because of the lack of education and limited experience with modern medicine the Kondh patients often make mistakes in the treatment procedure. Before taking a patient to the hospital, they try their ethno-medicine. In some cases, they may bring the patient to the hospital in a critical stage. So it becomes difficult for the doctor to treat such cases.

Most of the allopathic medicines have to be taken at specific intervals for checking the disease successfully. The tribals often make mistakes in taking the required dose of medicine in time. Sometimes when they go out for work, they may skip their doses. All these make the use of modern medicine ineffective.

Usually, the Kondhs are satisfied with a symptomatic relief and show much reluctance to come back to the hospital for continuing the treatment. This hesitation to visit the doctor for the follow-up treatment may prevent complete cure and lead to the return of the disease. An illness prolonging for a long time is considered as having originated due to the wrath of god.[40]

Kondhs are least bothered about following the advice of the doctor in respect of diet control, taking rest, avoiding hard work and smoking and drinking. They do not take rest unless they are so weak to do any work. Actually they do not know the relevance of these restrictions and their interrelationship with the treatment. The treatment is therefore not effective when the patient violates the advice of the doctor. Then the doctor and his medicines are considered as incapable of curing illness.

The shamans belonging to the community adopt a double standard in evaluating the efficacy of modern medicine in the treatment of diseases. Publicly they criticise modern medicine and opine that after curing one illness, it may cause another one. They also praise the advantages of ethno-medicine and explain to their clients, how it is suitable for the human body. They sometimes ridicule the folly of people, who seek modern medicine for the cure of illness.

But the strange fact is that when these shamans are affected by some diseases very often they go to the hospital or purchase medicine directly from the medicine shop. Often they try to hide from others that they are getting treatment from the hospitals. So they contact the doctors in the far away hospitals. This shows the double dealing of the shamans while evaluating the efficiency of modern medicine.[41]

The Kondhs are not aware of the relevance of preventive measures in the modern medicine for escaping from the diseases. They do not voluntarily take preventive injections for any disease. Some of them have got preventive injections as a part of the immunisation programmes of the government. But the people living in the remote areas are not often covered by these programmes. In their day-to-day life, they do not take any special care for the prevention of diseases. They have some supernatural measures like wearing of amulet, offering of sacrifices to god, etc., which are believed to be capable of preventing illnesses.

The Kondhs are not much aware of the relevance of personal hygiene and environmental sanitation in the prevention of diseases.

Most of them live in sub-human physical condition. Poor hygiene and polluted water spread a number of communicable and non-communicable diseases among them.[42] Actually they are not in a position to improve their living conditions due to socio-economic backwardness. When people do not have even the minimum necessities, it is hard for them to appreciate the value of preventive measures which will bring only probable benefits in the future. It is seen that in spite of visiting government doctors, tribal people have a great faith in their own system of medicine. Even though modern medicine was introduced in the tribal communities a number of decades ago, it has not yet attained the monopoly of health care among them. It plays only a complementary role along with ethno-medicine.

Shortage of sufficient number of doctors and qualified nurses is the greatest handicap of allopathic hospitals. The doctors and nurses are much reluctant to work in the tribal areas. After being posted in such places, they try to get a transfer from there as early as possible. Thus mere presence of a health centre is not enough. There may be health centres but without doctor and medicine.[43] Often the doctors do not come to the hospital regularly. The living conditions are very poor in the tribal areas and facilities of urban life are not there. Problems of housing, recreation, education of children and contact with the outside world are the common difficulties in such places.

Lack of adequate infrastructure is another hurdle facing modern medicine. In order to provide modern care services to the tribal people Primary Health Centres, dispensaries and hospitals have been established in tribal areas but the type of health care facilities they provide are not satisfactory. Health institutions in most of the tribal areas are understaffed.[44] There are no good buildings, beds, vehicles, laboratories, X-ray units and other essential equipments in the hospitals and Primary Health Centres functioning in the tribal areas. The doctors are much dissatisfied due to these adverse circumstances and sometimes they fail to diagnose the diseases correctly. These disadvantages adversely affect the quality of medical treatment available in these curative centres. Some of the doctors and medical staff complain that patient does not come to them but goes to their own healers viz, the magician, *gunias,* and such others. The patient continues to do so unless our doctors and paramedical personnel have a good knowledge about the tribal life, their culture and traditions and practices. Unless they understand their mental attitudes, their cultural beliefs, it is quite difficult on their part to make the government mission a successful one. They do not want to obtain health service from the government health agencies because of supply of sub-standard medicine and chronic problem of non-availability of required medicines. Health care service centres in the tribal areas are not coupled with quality service. That is why the death rate is high.[45] In these areas, there is lack of man power and the people are economically hand to mouth and they feel that without money treatment is not possible.

It is therefore the time to think seriously about the possibilities of micro level planning for health in tribal areas of Odisha. An integrated and inter-disciplinary approach to evolve suitable health programmes for different tribal communities is most desirable and constitutes an integral part of developmental programmes of the tribal communities of this state. The octopus of poverty is another hindrance for the success. It is very difficult to bring radical change. The prejudice of Kondh patients to accept wholly the modern medicine is also a hurdle, hindering its widespread recognition. The medicine men or shamans often resent modern medical programmes because they fear that the competition will be injurious to their status in the community.

Moreover, modernisation has significantly influenced their traditional knowledge, skill and technology. In their traditional lifestyle, direct and positive links between the traditional knowledge system and resource use are obvious. The knowledge pertaining to agriculture, forestry, healthcare and other fields is a valuable asset for the survival of the tribe. However things are changing in the method of treatment and choice of medicine. The more we are developing with the growth of science the more we are forgetting about the rich heritage and treasure. Though the Kondhs have faith on their own medicine, their inclination towards modern practice is developing.

The tribe is definitely in a transition between tradition and modernity. External programmes or policies intending to increase the efficiency of resource use so as to cope with increasing population pressure, scarcity and fluctuations in the environment or other contingencies require a blending of relevant formal and informal knowledge and institutions.[46]

In tribal system of health care, the medicine men or healers immensely use the plant and mineral based medicines for treatment of various kinds of illness. They are capable of demonstrating an amazing range of medical skills and expertise that extends from treating emergencies like poisonous bites to safe delivery, to cure asthma and other bronchial problems having complicated features. In thousands of villages where hardly any medical facility exists, they are the only source of support and hope for survival.[47] Tribal medicine has been evolved from the socio-cultural perceptional setups. These medicines are administered more as a means of preventing rather than curing diseases. Each indigenous tribal healer is recognised by the community as the most competent. He provide healthcare by using bio-resources, mineral substances and certain other methods, based on the socio-religious and cultural beliefs. These carriers of tribal health traditions have survived over thousands of years in spite of total lack of documentation and any institutional frame work to support and sustain them.

Modern medicine has come to stay among the tribes and it flourishes along with ethno-medicine which is still strong in the tribal world. Both play relevant roles in their health care and the tribals avail the facilities of the two systems with a sense of pragmatism. The ultimate aim of both systems of medicine is to preserve and protect the health of tribal people by fighting against different diseases. Total displacement of ethno-medicine will not be feasible at this stage and if attempted will be fatal to the tribals. In the ethno-medicine, there are certain components which would be retained because of their ecological and environmental advantages. Integration of modern medicine with the health habits of the tribals may appear simple and easily achievable but a number of ideological and practical hurdles are present in the way of attaining this goal. There is a need to integrate various systems of medicine existing among the Kondhs like ethno-botanical system, herbal medicine and allopathic system. A meaningful integration of the various systems would perhaps do a lot of good in improving physical, mental, social and emotional health of the tribals specially Kondhs. The community institutions like Kondh *Panchayat* and local leaders should be involved in coping up with various demands of the Kondh health, health planning service delivery and development.

There is certainly a need to preserve the age-old experienced practice of ethno-botanical knowledge potential as an indigenous alternative medicine which is accessible and cost effective simultaneously based on natural products without any side effects. In the developed world, more than 50 per cent of clinically useful drugs originate from natural sources. It is estimated that for

80 per cent of world population, plants play dominant role in their primary health care. It is realistic to expect that the entire population of the developing world will have access to modern medicine in the foreseeable future. However, great improvements in the health care can be achieved by systematisation of information about herbal medicine. About 16,000 flowering plants are available in India out of which 3,000 are recognised as used in ethno-medicine.[48]

The attitude of both doctors and medicine men has to be changed for attaining cooperation between these two systems of medicine. At present they have no common ground for meeting. Each looks at the other with suspicion. The modern physician additionally has contempt for ethno-medicine and this makes the tribals more suspicious of the doctors. A better understanding of each other's is essential for the development of such a friendly atmosphere. It is a common complaint of the health administrators that the tribals are not cooperating with them whenever they implement medical programmes for their benefit. But the administrators do not realise that this problem is arising due to lack of understanding about this new medical system. So imparting awareness among the tribals about modern medicine is an essential step for carrying out the medical programmes successfully.[49]

Studies on ethno-medicine ranges from paleopathology to recent times are within the sub fields of ethno-botany, folk medicine and medical anthropology.[50] Indigenous medicine is not contrary to the modern medicine rather it is very much complimentary. It has been proved that many indigenous methods have positive and beneficial effect. The indigenous systems are always autonomous system supported by the community, while allopathic drugs are only out reachable as well very expensive. Even today traditional medicine is known to cater to the health needs of more than 70 per cent of people in developing countries. World Health Organisation has given proper recognition to various indigenous systems of medicine for 'Global Health Care System', which is generally referred to as ethno-medicine. Ethno-medicine is a combination of those beliefs and practical relation to disease, which are products of indigenous cultural development. Nature has provided plant for every ailment and there is a cure for every disease and man has to find it out. When he faces health problem he takes the help of natural products of plants to cure diseases. Each tribe has its own system of indigenous health care practices based on local plant resources.[51]

New avenues must be opened to bring forth chances of better cooperation between the personnel of both systems of medicine. Such an understanding will be more useful for a modern medical practitioner. Then only he can interpret the behaviour of the tribal patients and understand why they are responding in a particular fashion on certain occasions. After getting a clear knowledge of their concepts of disease aetiology and healing, he can behave towards them in a better and more acceptable manner. Before attempting to work for a people we have to learn all about their way of life. There are three categories of treatments as ailments or sickness viz. (i) minor, (ii) medium and (iii) major, depending on the gravity of sufferings of patient. Minor ailments can be attended by trained health workers, the second category of sickness can be handled by general physician and the third category certainly requires the services of specialist physician/surgeons. If the literate tribal medicine men are imparted training in primary health care services then they can serve the tribal people in a better way and the present unwanted scene can be obviated. The suggestion needs to be debated and conclusions be arrived at. This sort of participatory development programmes will yield concrete and quick results and will be sustainable. It is time for identification and conservation of ethno-medicinal plants. Even more than half a century after independence our county is not yet developed in every sphere. Still the people are facing the problems of malnutrition and safe drinking water. Access to modern medical facilities for these persons is indeed a dream. Doctors and paramedical staff, all combined together cannot cater to the volume of basic health service of the tribal people of the state of Odisha. Therefore tribal and rural people continue to repose confidence on their traditional systems of medicine and medicine man. So it is desirable to train up the ethnic and traditional medicine man in fundamental allopathic systems of treatment for rendering better health care services to common masses. This sort of health care service will be participatory and sustainable in the long run.[52]

Since indigenous medicine is a social institution and an integral part of the tribal culture, that are included in a number of medical practices often employed in modern medicine. Simultaneously in the process of indigenous health care the medical beliefs, healing practices and medicine are crystallised in the form of ethno-scientific knowledge acquired by men. Therefore, the indigenous medical practices can be perpetuated as rational and efficacious methods. It is essential to document such languishing tradition. Hence, the tribal medicine and medicine men are to be safeguarded for their dedication to the suffering humanity. There is need for legal provision to protect the intellectual property rights under the General Agreement on Tariffs and Trade (GATT) and other allied international agreement. There is certainly a need to preserve the age old experienced practices of ethno-botanical knowledge potential as an indigenous alternative medicine, which is accessible and cost-effective.[53] When an existing body of knowledge is available, perhaps it is better to develop it instead of replacing it in the name of scientific development. World Health Organisation (WHO) has given good boost to the concept of integration of both the traditional and modern medicine.[54]

Since independence, India has been witnessing a ceaseless effort by government at the national as well as state level to deal with the problems of health which is vital to a county's all round development. A sizable portion of the nation's revenue is being spent on programmes of health and sanitation. As far as practicable, facilities have been extended to the remote corners of each state during the last five year plan period. The tribal development needs special and immediate attention of planners and administrators in general and anthropologists in particular. There is a need for co-ordination among administrators, anthropologists, government officials, planners, political leaders, social workers, tribal leaders and Non Government Organisation (NGO) workers.[55] In the villages, it is quite apparent that education is poor, other facilities like sanitation, drinking water, drainage, roads etc. are inadequate and the development of these facilities is not commensurate with the rural environment. Environmental education should be emphasised in the school curriculum. There is a dire need of programmes of health education among Kondhs to improve their health status.

It is quite often said that the rural people particularly the tribal communities, are generally reluctant to accept modern health practices. It is true that a number of deities are associated with particular diseases among many tribal communities of India and that tribals do worship a deity when there is illness in the family or community. When the tribals worship deity for cure automatically it is assumed that they are all superstitious but when the same thing is done in the city of Kolkata or Delhi or Mumbai or Chennai, it is tradition and when one prays to god for the cure of someone in a church of Europe or America, it is convention. This is how the same activity is differently labelled.[56]

While evaluating the overall effect of modern medicine upon the tribal community in general and ethno-medicine in particular, one can find that instead of competition or contradiction, there exists an atmosphere of coexistence and division of labour. The tribals employ their own pragmatism to decide what type of medicine must be used for a particular illness and use it accordingly. They resort to both ethno-medicine and modern medicine according to the aetiology and seriousness of different illnesses. So there is ample scope for the survival of both systems of medicine in the tribal universe. Each one deals with the type of disease for which it is found more effective. So in the present circumstances, both ethno and modern medical systems play a combined role in the health care of the tribals. The call of the hour is to make more scientific and comprehensive study to preserve the unique and valuable tribal knowledge treasure before it is completely lost.

References

1. Jose Boban K., *Tribal Ethnomedicine: Continuity and Change*, A.P.H. Publishing Corporation, New Delhi, 1998, 22.
2. *Ibid.*, 133.
3. B.L. Nagda, "Demographic Determinants of Tribal Health in Rajasthan", in Mohammad Akram, (ed.), *Health Dynamics and Margianalised Community*, Rawat Publication, New Delhi, 2007, 138.
4. N.K. Jha, "Our Ancient Wisdom", in Mohammad Akram, (ed.), *Health Dynamics and Margianalised Community*, Rawat Publication, New Delhi, 2007, 238.
5. Mitoo Das, "Disease and Illness and Their Ethonomedical Treatment Among the Rathwas of Suskal, Gujrat", A.K. Kalla and P.C. Joshi, (eds.) *Tribal Health and Medicine*, Concept Publishing Company, New Delhi, 2004, 283.
6. R.K. Kar, "Ethno Medicine and Tribal Health, An Illustrative Appraisal" in A.K. Kalla and P.C. Joshi, (eds.), *Tribal Health and Medicine*, Concept Publishing Company, New Delhi, 2004, 382-383.
7. Meena Gupta, "Neurological Disorders Among Tribals", in A. K. Kalla and P.C. Joshi, (eds.), *Tribal Health and Medicine*, Concept Publishing Company, New Delhi, 2004, 10.
8. Bijayalaxmi Dash and Nirmal Chandra Dash, *Kondhs, An Ethnobotanical Study,* Amadeus Press, Bhubaneswar, 2009, 27.

9. Robin D. Tribhuwan, *Medical World of Tribals*, Discovery Publishing House, New Delhi, 1998, 9.
10. G. Bulliya, *et al.*, "Indigenous Health Care Practice among the Kondh Tribal Communities of Orissa, India", in Awadesh N. Sharma, *et al.*, (eds.), *Indigenous Health Care and Ethnomedicine,* Sarup and Sons, New Delhi, 2006, 56.
11. N.K. Behura "Cultural Dimensions of Diseases and Their Treatment", *Adivasi,* Vol. XXXVII, No. 2, December 1997, Scheduled Castes and Scheduled Tribes Research and Training Institute (herein after SCSTRTI), Bhubaneswar, 11.
12. Sudipta Rath and P.K. Achrya, "Healing Practices of Tribal Medicinemen in Mayurbhananj District of Orissa", in *Adivasi*, Vol. 46, No. 1, June 2006, SCSTRTI, Bhubaneswar, 11.
13. Mihir Kumar Jena, Padmini Pathi, Kamala Kumari Patnaik and Klaus Seeland, *Forest Tribes of Orissa*, Vol. 2, *Kuttia Kondh*, D.K. Print World, New Delhi, 2006, 267.
14. N.K. Behura and K.K. Mohanti, *Tribal Orissa: Reading in Social Anthropology*, Dominant Publisher, New Delhi, 2006, 105-106.
15. Jose Boban K., *op. cit.*, 284-285.
16. *Ibid.*, 286.
17. Buddhadeb Chaudhuri, *Health, Forest and Development: the Tribal Situation*, Inter-India Publications, New Delhi, 2003, 38.
18. *Ibid.*, 40.
19. Jose Boban K., *op. cit.*, 2.
20. R.K. Kar, *op. cit.*, 388.
21. Buddhadeb Chaudhuri, *op. cit.,* 39.
22. G. Bulliyya, *et al.*, *op. cit.*, 63.
23. Mihir Kumar Jena, *et al., op. cit.,* 292.
24. Prasenjit Deb Burman, "Disease: Is it Individual or Societal"?, in Buddhadeb Chaudhuri, (ed.), *Tribal Health: Socio-cultural Dimensions*, Inter-India Publication, New Delhi, 1986, 185.
25. S.P. Gupta, "Tribal Concept of Health, Disease and Remedy", in Buddhadeb Chaudhuri, (ed.), *Tribal Health: Socio-cultural Dimension*, Inter-India Publications, New Delhi, 1986, 165.
26. Buddhadeb Chaudhuri, *op. cit.*, 44.
27. Jose Boban K., *op. cit.*, 296-297.

28. *Ibid.*, 298.
29. Buddhadeb Chaudhuri, *op. cit.*, 36-37.
30. *Ibid.*, 35.
31. Jose Boban K., *op. cit.*, 300- 301.
32. Buddhadeb Chaudhuri, *op. cit.,* 25.
33. Mihir Kumar Jena, *et al.*, *op. cit.*, 256.
34. A. K. Gamango, "Ethnic Healers among the Dongria Kondh of Orissa", *Advasi*, Vol. 47, No. 1 and 2, June and December, 2007, 149.
35. Jose Boban K., *op. cit.*, 270-271.
36. Pratap Kumar Singh, "Health Hazard in Tribal Societies of Orissa and its Remedy" in Jyotsna Mohanty, (ed.), *Tribal Health, Culture and Development in Orissa,* Kamala Nehuru College, Bhubaneswar, 2004, 181.
37. *Ibid.*, 180.
38. Jose Boban K., *op. cit.*, 276.
39. *Ibid.*, 279.
40. *Ibid.*, 280.
41. *Ibid.*, 281.
42. G. Bulliyya, *et al.*, *op. cit.*, 60.
43. Buddhadeb Chaudhuri, *op. cit.,* 25.
44. N.K. Behura and K. K. Mohanty, *op. cit.*, 140.
45. Pratap Kumar Singh, *op. cit.,* 181.
46. Mihir Kumar Jena, *Kuttia Kondh*, *op. cit.*, 293.
47. Sudipta Rath and P. K. Acharya, "Health Practices of Tribal Medicinemen in Mayurbhanj District of Orissa", *Adivasi*, Vol. 46, No. 1, June, 2006, SCSTRTI, 11.
48. G. Bulliyya, *et al.*, *op. cit.*, 55.
49. Jose Boban K., *op. cit.*, 300.
50. G. Bulliyya, *et al.*, *op. cit.*, 55.
51. *Ibid.,* 56.
52. N.K. Behura and K.K. Mohanty, *op. cit.*, 140-141.
53. G. Bulliyya, *et al.*, *op. cit.*, 63.
54. B. Sanjeev Reddy, "An Approach to the Integration of Traditional Medicine and Modern Medicine: A Hypothetical Model" in Buddhadeb Choudhury, (ed.), *Tribal Health: Socio-*

cultural Dimensions, Inter-India Publications, New Delhi, 1986, 23.

55. Pramod Mishra, *Ecology, Culture and Health of a Primitive Tribe*, Serials Publication, New Delhi, 2004, 311.
56. Buddhadeb Chaudhuri, *op. cit.*, 45.

Conclusion

Odisha occupies an unparallel position in the ethnographic map of India for having the largest number of *adivasi* groups or aboriginal/tribal communities. Each community has its own cultural identity and distinctiveness in terms of tradition, social organisation, customs, language, rituals, festivals, dress, ornaments, art and craft. Out of sixty-two tribal communities that inhabit the state, Kondhs are numerically the largest and the seventh largest tribe in India. They are one of the major primitive tribes of India, are older than the Vedic Aryans and even the Dravidian architect of the ancient Indian civilisation. Geographically isolated, socially, educationally and economically backward, Kondhs continue to live in dense forests, hills and inaccessible areas of the state, mostly in southern part of Odisha. They still lead a simple, traditional and colourful life in valleys and lush forests under primitive situation and insalubrious climate, maintaining their independence and preserving their indigenous language, animistic religion, customs and traditions.

Living in this primitive condition for centuries together and keeping themselves in isolation, most of the Kondhs are unaware of so-called modern civilisation and the rapid changes that have been taking place in other places particularly in plains. Like all other tribal communities, Kondhs are also famous for their magnificent typical cultural heritage and they still cherish old tribal traditions and concepts. Their ways of living with minimum needs of food, shelter and clothing seem to have remained unaltered or a little changed through the centuries. The sacred god-nature-man relationship that works among them is an amazing experience to the mind of modern man. Kondhs are classified into three sub groups, viz., Desia, Kutia and Dongria. Desia Kondhs are different from Kutia and Dongria Kondhs. Kutias and Dongrias still maintain strong individual identity and cultural status. In contrast, Desias have been exposed to modernity because of their frequent interaction with the non-tribal people of plains. They are the most advanced section and inhabit the plain areas.

Kondhs consider themselves as the original inhabitants of the soil. Their way of life is based on their ability to utilise the available natural resources to the maximum in order to attain self sufficiency. Forests are intimately connected with Kondh life and economy. To vast majority of the Kondh people, the forest is their well-loved home, their livelihood, and their very existence depends on forests. Since time immemorial, they have been enjoying the freedom to use forest products or hunt animals and this has given them a conviction that the forest belongs to them. The forest is the main source of livelihood of these people. Their economy is by and large based on activities around the jungles. Food gathering and haunting continue to be the main source of livelihood, though some of the Kondh people have become agriculturists. They are born in forest, live in forest and die in forest. Their socio-cultural as well as economic umbilical cord is attached to the nature- the forest and the hills. In a nutshell, they are permanently indebted to forest.

Kondhs are simple, well-manned, faithful, generous, polite and hospitable. They are also known for their remarkable fidelity and valour. They have a great respect for their social customs such as birth, marriage and death, the three great incidents of life. They have their distinct identity, which is marked in their social organisations, language, rituals, festivals, dress, ornament, art and, craft, beliefs, treatment of disease and lifestyle. These things descended from antiquity have been preserved till date. On the other hand nature has taught them to love, respect, fear and worship the forces of nature. Each sex group sticks to its work as per social sanctions. Women are very hard working and do all sorts of work from dawn to dusk. They live in a caste-free society and that gives each person the freedom to experience, touch, smell, see and hear all aspects of the forest and its products.

The cycle of life offers them numerous reasons to celebrate every moment with vigour and grace either in privacy of family or in community as a whole. The birth of a child, marriage, death, etc. is observed family-wise. On the other hand cultivation, hunting etc. are observed as community or village ceremonies. The changing seasons, religious customs and the traditional rhythms of superstitious belief are strong incentives for creating a string of festivals to be celebrated by them. In spite of poverty and other constraints, they have managed to retain their rich and diverse heritage. They observe a number of festivals and worship different gods and goddesses to prevent and cure diseases. They relate their dreams to some of the events of the life to be happened in the near future. This speaks clearly their inclination for their culture and faith.

An enquiry into the world of a tribal community of Odisha means to explore a society closely interlinked to the natural and spiritual space that constitutes its habitat. Kondh myths, rituals and customs have been developed from their natural environment while the worship of animate and inanimate elements indicates their love and fear of nature. It is a common observation among these people that ancestral spirits play an important role in the prosperity and protection of the family. Hence they have to be properly honoured otherwise they will bring wrath on family members. These spirits are believed to bring a state of physical, mental and social well-being to the members of the family. On the other hand there are many spirits who are feared because of their power to afflict people by brining number of diseases. Sickness is not natural to Kondh people. It is due to machination of some evil spirits or indignation of ancestor spirits or gods. To them sickness is considered as the consequences of certain lapses on the part of individual or community as a whole and the remedy must be sought through propitiation and observance of rituals. Kondhs also believe that men, animals, birds, reptiles and plants co-exist in symbolic relationship. Any disturbance in this relationship can bring disastrous outcome. The fear of the environment has made Kondhs extremely superstitious. They believe that the unusual occurrence in nature or the events of life are caused by deities or other supernatural powers. So they appease these powers by sacrifice. They are used to practice many superstitious customs because they have a strong belief in magic, sorcery and witchcraft.

The religious beliefs and practices of Kondh people are curious combination of animism, nature worship, shamanism and ancestor worship. These practices seek to ensure personal security and happiness as well as the community well being and unity. They are more influenced by socio-cultural and environmental dimensions in their healing practices. Since they associate sickness, death and good health with the blessing or curse of the deities worshipped by them, appeasement of gods and goddesses form the major part of their belief system concerning health care. While conducting rituals, the shamans act as diviners and astrologers. A piece of stone, a trunk of tree or even thatched structures are objects of worship. For them, animal sacrifice and liquor are vital ingredients. They believe in observing totemic rites, taboos and special rituals for invoking rain and elimination of diseases.

Their magico-religious performances are associated with several types of sacrifices and observances. It needs blood of animals and birds starting from a pigeon to buffaloes. Most of their magico-religious performance are followed by music, dance and drinking. They worship specific gods and goddesses and perform certain special rituals to prevent and cure different diseases. A ritual like *Puchana* is conducted by the shaman to diagnose the cause of disease whereas. *Lodang* is usually conducted by these people after getting cured. *Badabiha Dakina* is observed to cure any serious disease. To prevent chickenpox and cholera they observe *Ghanta Parba*. *Siruki Bakada* is observed to protect the unborn child in the mother's womb. *Eju Penu Dakina* is a ritual conducted to cure diseases caused by evil spirit. As they believe the medicinal plants are the real treasure to save life they observe a special ritual called *Asa Dakina* which is otherwise known as medicinal plant worship. Beliefs and practices concerning life cycle, agricultural operation, house construction, food gathering and haunting are some of the special features of the Kondh magico-religious activities.

The concept of health is understood more in functional terms than clinical among the Kondhs. Their health is related to environment, habitat, and socio-cultural and magico-religious beliefs. Kondhs attach more importance to other aspects of life but not to health. They are not aware of the fact that health is the most precious aspect of life and negligence of health adversely affects all aspects of development of the individual. Kondhs still have a very strong faith in their ethno-medical practices. This is because most of them are forest dwellers and are shy of social contacts. They are unable to spend adequately on food and clothing. They do not bother about hygiene and environmental sanitation.

The wide spread poverty, illiteracy, malnutrition, absence of safe drinking water, unhygienic and insanitary living conditions, poor maternal and child care health services, ineffective coverage of National Health and Nutritional Services are factors for dismal health conditions prevailing among these people. All living beings in a fundamental sense depend on three basic life-support materials viz. air, water and food for their survival. But the Kondhs are totally less concerned about these three components. They are deprived of basic amenities of life but in spite of that they lead a content life. The protein content in their food is insignificant as they depend on the forests and domestic animals for their food. They are also unable to supplement their diet with milk or pulses. Besides this, they get very little vitamin from their diet. Above all semi-starvation, inferior diet and unhygienic living condition attribute to the prevalence of number of diseases like nutritional and metabolic disorders, dysentery, diarrhoea, fever, asthma, etc. The skin diseases are very common among Kondhs. Heavy alcohol drinking with insufficient diet causes gastric, colic and dyspepsia and tuberculosis. Besides this, most of them are affected by malaria. Sporadic cases of cholera are also there in Kondh areas. They not only suffer from a number of diseases but also maternal and child mortality rate are high amongst these people. Many factors such as inadequate diet intake of mothers, low birth weight of baby, labour complications, inadequate supplementary feeding and lack of immunisation are also responsible for this.

The treatment of the disease is usually conducted through propitiation of the deities according to the prescription of their medicine man. Kondhs come to the doctors at the last stage of the disease or disability after all their attempts to appease the spirits failed. At this stage, it becomes difficult on the part of the doctor to cure the patient. Costly life saving drugs required in acute cases is not often available in hospitals and they are unable to purchase drugs due to their poor economic condition. This community is away from the mainstream of civilisation and lacks medical facilities curative as well as preventive. As per their belief, they suffer and die when they cannot appease the 'angry spirit' and fail to get divine blessings.

Although a large number of plants are associated with their food, economy and religion, the use of plant species for medicinal purposes is surprisingly more. Even where the Kondhs are having government health care centres, the services of the *disari, kutaka* and *jani* for traditional medicine among them is quite remarkable. This is due to easy availability of traditional system of cure and its cost effectiveness. If medicine is a social institution as per Encyclopaedia of Social Sciences then a medicine man is an office bearer in the society. The medicine man possesses a comprehensive knowledge about the medicinal plants, herbs, tubers, roots, barks, leaves, flowers, seeds, fruits, birds, reptiles and animals in their environment from which medicines are manufactured and administered. The indigenous knowledge of the Kondhs on medicinal plants plays a vital role in their primary health care since the hoary past.

Plants play a pivotal role in the life of Kondhs. They are the real custodian of medicinal plants. This ethnic tribal community inhabiting in thick and dense forest possesses rich knowledge about plant wealth. As they are living close to nature, they have acquired unique knowledge of living plant resources over the years. This knowledge has been gathered and transmitted orally through generations. They use a large number of plants and plant products in the treatment of different ailments. The most commonly used plants are: *Harida, Bahada, Amla, Tulasi, Bela, Basanga, Indramarisa, Nimba, Odisamari, Asoka, Arakha, Bhuinimba, Dimbiri, Hadabhanga Jada, Kaincha, Kalara, Babulla, Bisalyakarani, Brahmi,* etc.

They usually depend on herbal medicines in case of general sickness and in serious cases only they attend medical dispensaries. Ethno-botany is the interdisciplinary scientific study of interaction between plants and people since time immemorial. In fact a number of ethno-botanical studies have helped to identify a number of medicinal plants used by this tribal community to treat different types of diseases. Many of them may be very useful and it is urgently necessary to document them and try them after proper scientific experiment. In a pluri-medicinal country like that of ours there is need for the promotion of ethno-medicine which is practiced by these people. The system of ethno-medicine is participatory and cost effective. The rich and untapped flora which Kondhs have been using for food and medicine required to be studied. They represent an invaluable indigenous knowledge base which needs to be documented. Their traditional understanding of plant resources can help the mankind to find out the ecological inter-relations which even the modern ecologists and plant scientists would find difficult. The ethno-medical knowledge of the tribal people will be helpful to prepare clinical useful compounds from plant resources. The World Health Organisation has been promoting a movement for "saving plants for saving lives." This is because of the growing understanding of the vital role medicinal plants play in providing herbal remedy for health maladies. Hence there is an urgent need of forest management, which will be helpful for the conservation of many endangered plant species that are on the verge of extinction.

It is observed that Kondh societies have been changing at a certain pace in terms of their health seeking behaviour. The rapid depletion of natural surroundings and ecosystem compounded with infiltration and intrusion of non-tribal elements into tribal domain play a major role in changing Kondh culture, value system and their world view. The study certainly points out that the traditional health care system still finds its meaning of survival in tribal domain. The traditional medicine man who is considered as the guardian of tribal society acts as the medium between man on the one hand and nature, supernatural entity on the other hand. He provides spiritual security to the tribal people. This is the link on which the uniqueness of tribal society exists. The Kondhs feel secured with protection given by their traditional medicine men against psycho-social problems or spiritual insecurity. But it is seen that many government policies hardly accept this component in their health related aids and campaigns. A rational synthesis of traditional perceptions with modern facilities would certainly give better results in tribal health issues and their solution.

The great dilemma in health seeking behaviour that often a Kondh individual faces is the choice that he has to make between custom bound practices and beliefs which are laden with socio-religious values and the modern system which is projected as better than the other by the people who are often strangers. Indeed Kondhs are in a transitional phase of going away from the ethno-medicine and indigenous methods of treatment and half-hearted acceptance of modern system of medical care and treatment. The tribal patient will continue to do so unless our doctors and paramedical staff have a good knowledge about these people, their culture and traditions, customs and practices. They should understand the constraints such as their mental attitude and deep rooted cultural belief, poverty, communication barrier, geographical isolation, etc., which prevent them from taking the advantage of existing health services. So any plan to provide health care to these tribal communities has to reckon with few basic realities of the tribal life. In order to convince them we must give healing touch and a lot of patience is required for it, then only it will be fruitful.

Their health needs special and immediate attention. It demands an integrated approach to improve their economic, educational and hygienic conditions. They are economically hand to mouth. The present day medical treatment is a costly affair. Due to weak economic condition and lack of rational knowledge, the Kondhs never get the blessings of modern medicine for severe ailments. Hence they rush to their local healers for curing illness. People cannot save the lives of serious patients due to their emotional beliefs on the village and religious functionaries. It is therefore time to look into seriously the possibilities of micro level planning for health in these areas of Odisha. An integrated and interdisciplinary approach to evolve suitable health programmes for different tribal communities including the Kondhs is most desirable at this point of time.

These tribal people are to be educated about the value of health and hygiene and importance of medical care. In contrast to traditional health care system, the official health care system is based on modern science and technology separating it from broader social and cultural concerns and influences. It is evident that state supported modern medical system does not generally recognise the traditional medical system. Several studies have proved that traditional societies do not get the most needed psychological security in modern medical system as it ignores the cultural components of disease and treatment prevailing in a given society. Only the policies of the government cannot wash out all the tribal problems. It needs proper planning. Development of a group or an area can be possible with due emphasis on their traditional values and historical experiences.

One could see the real impact of modernity on the tribal society in general and the Kondhs in particular. With the march of time, it is quite difficult on their part to remain separate and maintain their proverbial exclusiveness. Tribes including Kondhs responded to intrusion, administrative as well as cultural, of the non-tribal people in different ways. The distance between the tribal people and other communities has decreased apparently. The benefits of the modern civilisations in the fields of education, communication, agriculture, transport, health care, etc. should be made available to the tribal people including the Kondhs but not at the cost of their culture retained so far. Being the people of so called modern civilisation, when we are following our tradition that we learn from our ancestors, we cannot reject their beliefs and practices which are dear to them than their life.

The cultural heritage of Kondhs is intricately interwoven with various cultural activities, beliefs and practices. In a changing canvas, Kondhs have been able to retain their identity to perpetuate their way of life because of their cultural apparatus. Their age old and rich cultural heritage has been responsible for the maintenance of self identity. Despite the impact of modern civilisation, they strive hard for retention and replenishment of their traditional culture which is reflected through their manners, customs, beliefs, rituals, ethos, ideologies, values, norms, ethics, dance, songs, music, art and crafts, recreation and leisure . These societies are valuable parts of our national heritage. They must develop in every sphere and share in the growing national prosperity and contribute to it. At the same time, as they develop and modernise, care must be taken to see that they do not lose those precious aspects of their culture and life.

Glossary

Technical Terms used by Kondhs

Akinga	:	Fermented liquor made from mahua
Aku Saritei	:	Environment
Amba Kalu	:	Mango liquor
Arkhi Kalu	:	Mahua liquor
Bada	:	Adjacent to cultivated land
Baila	:	One type of pulses
Bajanidu	:	Kitchen
Bedana roga	:	Sexually transmitted disease
Beju	:	The Shaman who is specialist in divination
Bejuni	:	The Shamanin who is specialist in divination
Bhata	:	One type of fertile land
Bichhu mara	:	A special herb sprang up first by god for Kondhs

Bidi	:	Tobacco rolled in kendu leaves used for smoking
Bidi mara	:	One type of herb having medicinal value
Boda	:	Sacrifice of a goat
Bodokoocha	:	Plant that sprang up first in earth by God
Boora penu	:	Sun God
Brapa numberi	:	Malaria
Chati	:	Mushroom
Chilimati	:	One type of clay Kondhs use to clean hair
Chunga	:	One type of local cigar
Dadi	:	Fever
Dadu	:	Ring worm
Dahi cultivation	:	A type of cultivation in which the land is ploughed with the help of cattle
Danginpdika	:	Ascariasis
Dapanidu	:	Bed room
Deukuda	:	Village God
Dhangadabasa	:	Boys' dormitory
Dhangadibasa	:	Girls' dormitory
Dhapa	:	Small room near first room
Dharmadevata	:	Lord of Justice
Dhongla	:	One type of narcotic
Dinda Ghara	:	Girl's dormitory
Disari	:	Medicine man of Kondhs
Dongar	:	Hill slope land for shifting cultivation
Dua	:	Raw tobacco
Duma or Dumba	:	Spirit
Duri kalu	:	Rice or ragi kalu
Eja	:	Home
Gada	:	Medicine
Gaheli	:	Shed
Ghanta	:	Earthen pot
Guda kalu	:	Molasses liquor

Gundru	:	One type of bird
Gunia	:	Magician who believes on the efficacy of mantra vidya
Hapna	:	Dream
Hate	:	Death
Ichha Jani	:	Assistant of Jani who arranges the rituals
Ilu	:	House
Irpi-kalu	:	Mahua liquor
Jada	:	Forest
Jaka	:	A separate enclosure in the house
Jani	:	Ritual head of the kondh village
Janniyani	:	Village priestes
Jantal	:	When Kondhs sacrificed goat or cock instead of buffalo the name of Kedu festival replaced by another name called as Jantal
Jatrakudi	:	Village Goddess or deity
Jella	:	Life/Soul
Jhudunga	:	One type of pulses
Jiu or Jurma	:	Life
Joda Kayu	:	Wild fowl
Kadali kalu	:	Plantain liquor
Kaji	:	Eye-shoot to escape from evil eye
Kaju	:	Jungle fowl
Kalu	:	Wine
Kandha	:	Inhabitants of the hills.
Kandula	:	Red gram
Kane	:	Leprosy
Kapadabisa	:	Headache
Kara	:	One type of narcotic
Kara mara	:	One type of plant or herb used for medicine
Kata Mahane or Ekla Mahane	:	A place of burial for women who die during pregnancy/children who die within 4 to 5 years of age.
Kating	:	One type of pulses

Katuli	: Fermented liquor made from one kind of millet
Kedu	: When Kondhs sacrificed buffalo instead of human being the name of meriah festival has been replaced by another name called kedu.
Khada	: Pith of spinach
Khajuri Kalu	: Date-palm juice (liquor)
Khati	: Malevolent spirit
Kirang	: Parrot
Kolali	: Mahua or Salap liquor.
Konda	: Hill
Kondas	: Hill men
Kuchha	: Leaves or spinach
Kuda	: Clan
Kudeli	: A hut where Dharani Penu is installed
Kugure	: Dove
Kuguria	: One type of bird
Kui	: Kondh language
Kui Enju	: Kondh people
Kui lok	: Kondh people
Kuinga	: Plural form of kui.
Kumbhatal	: One type of bird
Kundeli	: One type of narcotic
Kutaka	: The sorceror in Kutia kondh society
Kuti	: Cave
Linga	: Human body made up of clay
Losom	: Cold
Mada kalu or Madanga	: Sago-palm liquor
Mahane	: Ghost
Mahua	: Mahula
Mala	: Hill tracts.
Mantra	: Magical spell

Marlu	:	Rabbit
Meriah	:	Victim of human sacrifice.
Meriah parb	:	Festival observed for good harvest in which human being is sacrificed
Milu	:	Peacock
Munda	:	Post
Mungugiri ejce	:	Rhinitis
Mutha	:	Bigger unit than clan
Nangal kanda	:	One type of tuber
Nemberi	:	Fever
Neripata	:	Blood dysentery
Niyama Raja	:	A mythical king
Nomberi	:	Fever
Pada	:	Mantra (Magical spell)
Padomba	:	Evil spirit causes cough and cold fever
Pali nomberi	:	Fever
Panasa Kalu	:	Jack fruit liquor
Pandka	:	Pigeon
Pano	:	A low caste Hindu
Pat Bejuni	:	Elder Bejuni
Patadai		Diarrhoea
Pataklipangene	:	Amoebic dysentery
Patobish	:	Stomach disease
Penu	:	God
Petpur	:	Heaven
Pika	:	Local cigar made of leaves
Pitatuste	:	Abortion
Poda	:	Buffalo
Podu	:	Shifting cultivation
Pranga akinga	:	Rice beer
Pua	:	A cylindrical stone-roller-pin
Puchuna	:	A ritual to diagnosis disease.
Pujari	:	Priest

Pulto Bagho	:	Kondhs tranform themselves into tigers by magic called pulto Bagho
Punja	:	Larger agnatic descent group
Raga mara	:	A special herb sprang up first by God for Kondhs
Rangakoocha	:	Kondhs believe that it is a plant which sprang up first in earth by God
Ranikanda	:	One type of tuber
Rohu fish	:	A special type of fish
Sadar	:	Community
Salpa	:	Juice from salpa tree
Sari	:	Myna
Sechkanti	:	Vomiting
Senju	:	Scabics
Sila	:	Flat rectangular stone base
Sisa	:	Assistant to Disari
Sranki	:	Porcupine
Tabala	:	Amulets
Tambi	:	A wooden or metal measure
Tambi	:	One and half kilogram or more
Tanha	:	Cough
Terka	:	Bamboo shoot
Thakurani	:	Mother Goddess
Topari	:	One type of narcotic
Tuli munda	:	Wooden post in the upper part of the Kondh hut
Ukodi	:	Soul

Appendix-I

Medicinal Plants in Use

As Identified by Khonds	*Commonly Used Names*	*Botanical Names*
Agara	Odisamari	Argemone mexicana
Agasti	Agasthi	Sesbania grandiflora
Alu	Alu kanda	Solanum tuberosum
Ambilasag	Ambiliti	Oxalis carniculata
Ambrut	Amruta bhanda	Carica Papaya
Ankuranti	Ankranti	Solanum xanthocarpum
Aparajita	Aparajita	Cliteria ternatea
Arak mara	Arakha	Calotropis gigantea
Arguna	Aruna	Cycas circinalis
Asuda	Asadua	Capparis zeylanica
Atkir	Muturi	Smilax zeglanica
Babui Tulsi	Dahana	Ocimum basilicum
Babur	Babulla	Acacia nilotica

As Identified by Khonds	*Commonly Used Names*	*Botanical Names*
Badalimba	Mahanimba	Melia azedarach
Baena mara	Bahada	Terminalia bellirica
Baidimiri	Dimbiri	Ficus racemosa
Baila	Baila	Lablab purpureus
Baincha	Baincha	Flacourtia cataphracta
Bana bhalia	Bhalia	Semecarpus anacardium
Bariar	Bajramuli	Sida cordata
Basango	Basanga	Jasticia adhatoda
Belamara	Bela	Aegle marmelos
Chandana	Chandana	Santalum album
Chhedabay	Patalgaruda	Rauvolfia serpentina
Chiramar or Sugandhi	Ananta mula	Hemidesmus indicus
Dhala Ankola	Ankula	Alangium salvifolium
Dhamana mara	Dhamana	Grewia tilifolia
Dhau	Dhou	Anogeissus latifolia
Dudhi	Dudhi	Cryptolepis buchananii
Dudhkadi	Dudhilata	Oxystelma esculanta
Dudura	Kaladudura	Datura metel
Dundi	Hinjala	Barringtonia acutangula
Gachcho Janaya	Malanga	Vanda tessellate
Gaigaruda	Gaigobaria	Costus speiosus
Gambar mara	Gambhari	Gmelina arborea
Gandhuli	Prasaruni	Paederia foetida
Gheekuanri	Ghee Kuanri	Aloe-vera
Giredi	Bada Gilo	Entada pursaetha
Gohira	Kantasarisa	Acacia leucophloea
Golakanta	Kantasaru	Lasia spinosa
Golamaricha	Golamaricha	Piper nigrum
Gursilai	Guluchilata	Tinospora cordifolia

As Identified by Khonds	*Commonly Used Names*	*Botanical Names*
Had Bhanga	Hada Bhanga	Cissus quadrangula
Hasasanga	Konda alu	Deoscorea belophylla
Hid	Piasal	Pterocarpus marsupium
Hinga	Haladi	Curcuma longa
Irpi mara	Mahula	Madhuca indica
Jamu mara	Pijuli	Psidium guajava
Jambu mara	Jamukoli	Syzygium cumini
Jangali Kaniyari	Koniyari	Cascabela thevetia
Jhajangi	Jhanjika	Breynia rhamnoides
Jida	Jida	Ficus microcarpa
Jomai Kaice	Chakunda	Cassia tora
Kaanga	Harada	Cajanus cajan
Kabang	Jada	Ricinus communis
Kadki	Tandi	Sacecharum spentaneum
Kaith	Kaitha	Limonaa acidissima
Kalchia	Kalchua	Glochidion zeylanicum
Kalmeg	Bhui nimba	Andrographis paniculata
Kamilimarmu	Barun	Crateva magna
Kanda koli	Kerenda koli	Carissa carandas
Kanikanta	Koilekha	Hygrophila auriculata
Kantaneutia	Kantaleutia	Amaranthus spinosus
Kara	Kachila khai	Strychnos nux-vomica
Kattapeng	Pengu	Pavetta tomentosa
Kaunria saga	Khata Palanga	Hibiscus sabdariffa
Kendumara	Kendu	Diospyros melanoxylon
Kenua	Pitakeruan	Holarrhena pubescens
Kojari	Khajuri	Phoenix Sylvestris
Kolthia	Bana Kolthia	Atylosia scarabaeoides
Kosaikoli	Kaseikoli	Diospyrous chloroxylon

As Identified by Khonds	*Commonly Used Names*	*Botanical Names*
Kubabal	Nagarjuna	Leucaena leucocephala
Kulthia	Banakolathia	Tephrosia maxima
Kumbre	Kumbhi	Careya arborea
Kundoru	Dantari kanta	Acacia pennata
Kuyan	Alasi	Guizotia abyssinica
Lajuli	Lajakuli	Mimosa pudica
Lalchita	Lalchitaparu	Plumbago indica
Lankanal	Baigaba	Jatropha gossypifolia
Leka mara	Simili	Bombax ceiba
Leli mara	Tentuli	Tamarindus indica
Lembu	Lembu	Citrus aurantifelia
Lenguli mara	Bichhuati	Laportea interrupta
Lipalu	Shiju	Cerus pteroynas
Mada mara	Salopo	Caryota urens
Madang	Malang	Scurrula parasitica
Madarangasaga	Madaranga	Alternanthera sessilis
Mandara	Mandar	Hitriscus rosa sinensis
Mardang	Karada	Cleistanthus collinus
Masania	Masani	Aporosa octandra
Maska mara	Amba	Mangifera indica
Masu	Sissoo	Dalbergia latifolia
Meral	Kontaikoli	Firmiana indica
Mukta manji	Ritha	Sapindus emarginata
Muruga	Lurga	Sansevieria roxburghiana
Musakani Nai	Musakani	Ipomoea sepiaria
Naktichana	Indramarisa	Acalypha indica
Nanam	Mohi	Lannea coromandelica
Nilkain	Nilakain	Nymphaea nouchali
Nima mara	Nimba	Azadirachta indica
Nirgundi	Begunia	Vitex nigundo

As Identified by Khonds	*Commonly Used Names*	*Botanical Names*
Palasa	Palash	Butea monosperma
Panasa	Panasa	Artocarpus heterophyllus
Parsia	Phansi	Anogeissus acuminata
Penhepari	Satabari	Asparagus racemosus
Pichubara	Barada	Bauhinia purpurea
Pipada mara	Jari	Ficus scandens
Pitakanda	Pitakanda	Doscorea bulbifera
Pitana	Kochila	Strychos nux vomica
Pithalakanda	Panialu	Dioscorea oppositifolia
Podam	Kadmba	Neolamarckia cadamba
Rakṭa Pitchali	Khanta	Gouania leptostachya
Ramkedar	Bano Ada	Zingiber purpurem
Rani kuna	Kandamula	Ipomoea batatas
Relu	Gilo	Caesalpinia diyyna
Reri/ Giridi	Giridi	Casearia graveolens
Rola	Harida	Terminalia chebula
Runja	Kainch	Abrus precatorius
Rusabodu	Apamaranga	Achyranthes aspera
Salimba	Saliabanso	Dendno calamus strictus
Sangel Sali	Bheru	Chloroxylon swietiana
Sanjam	Sal	Shorea robusta
Sara	Sahada	Streblus asper
Sarsakucha	Sonsa	Brassica Juncea
Saru	Sarukanda	Colocasia esculenta
Sehar	Siali	Bauhini vahlii
Sembed	Paladhua	Erythrina variegata .
Sidyce	Siriso	Albizia lebbeck
Siju	Dokanasiju	Euphorbia antiquorum
Sirisan	Dhalasirisa	Albicia procera

As Identified by Khonds	*Commonly Used Names*	*Botanical Names*
Sitaparu	Dhala chitaparu	Plumbago zeylanica
Sitaphala	Sitaphala	Annona Squamosa
Subudhibarso	Akanbindhi	Cissampelos Pareira
Sunderi mara	Sunari	Cassia fistula
Surgamara	Amla	Phyllanthus embilica
Tadi	Kadali	Musa paradisiaca
Tingan	Kongra	Xylia xylocarpa
Tungam Sanga	Pita alu	Dioscorea wallichie
Tutudu	Tuttudi kanta	Canthium parviflorum
Urla	Pokasunga	Ageratum conyzoides
Usangid	Ashok	Saraca asoca
Yarromaddi	Arjuna	Terminalia arjuna

APPENDIX-II

Questionnaire

1. What is your view about health and disease?
2. What is your view about belief?
3. What are the common diseases you suffer from?
4. What is your view about hygiene?
5. What is the role of *Jani/Disari/Kutaka*?
6. What is your view about herbal medicine?
7. Which plants do you use?
8. Do you use medicinal plants for the purpose of medicine only?
9. Which parts do you use root/stem/leaf/juice/flower?
10. For preparation of medicine which ingredients do you add to it?
11. Application of medicine, whether oral or external?
12. To what extent diseases get cured?
13. Success percentage?
14. Local medicine or modern medicine, which do you prefer?

15. In case of failure of local medicines what do you do?
16. Is your weak economic condition an obstacle for the use of modern medicine?
17. What is your view about surgery?
18. Do you think traditional method of treatment is better than modern method?
19. Where the Public Health Centre on your area located?
20. What is the distance to PHC from your village?
21. What is the mode of transport?
22. Have you ever gone to PHC Dispensary/Hospital for treatment? Yes/No
23. Have you availed the facilities in PHC Dispensaries/Hospitals? Yes/No
24. When your family member becomes ill, to whom you go for treatment first? *Jani*/ *Gunia*/ Doctor
25. What difficulties do you face while availing services from Health centres
    (a) Loss of wage
    (b) Long distance
    (c) No proper convenience
    (d) No satisfactory health care
    (e) Any other
26. What do you think when a person becomes ill?
    (a) Due to physical disorder
    (b) Due to wrath of evil spirit
    (c) Any other factors

Bibliography

I. Primary Sources

(i) Selections from Government Records and Reports

Selection from the Records of Ganjam Collectorate, 1842, Chatrapur, 1936.

Selections from the Old Records of Ganjam Collectorate, 1840, Chatrapur, 1935.

Selections from the Old Records of the Madras Government, No. XXIV, Madras, 1856.

Selections from the Records of Bengal Government, No. III, Calcutta, 1867.

(ii) Reports and Correspondences

Ali, Almas, (Special Officer on Tribal Health), *Health and Nutritional Profiles of Tribal Villages of Orissa*, Unpublished Report, Scheduled Castes and Scheduled Tribes Research and Training Institute (SCSTRTI), Bhubaneswar, 1980.

Ali, Almas, *Report on Health and Genetic Problems of Kutia Khonds of Burlubaru Village, Phulbani District*, Orissa, Tribal and Harijan Research cum Training Institute (THRTI) and Tribal and Rural Welfare Department (TRW), Bhubaneswar, 1979.

Basu, S.K. and Anil Jindal, *Report on Genetic and Socio-cultural Dimension of Tribal Health, A Primitive Kutia Kondh, Tribal Group of Phulbani District, Orissa*, New Delhi, Indian Council of Medical Research (ICMR) Project, 1990.

Campbell, John, *Report on Ghoomsur in Ganjam*, 1942.

Macpherson, John, *Report on* the *Kondhs of Ganjam and Cuttack Districts,* 1863.

Macpherson, S.C., *Report on the Human Sacrifice of the Kondhs*, 1841.

Patnaik, N., Almas, Ali. Ch., Prasanta K. Mahapatra and K. B. Debi, *Report on A Preliminary Health Survey in Four Tribal Blocks of Orissa*, Bhubaneswar, 1981.

Patnaik, N. and Almas Ali, *Report on Study of Health and Nutritional Status of Tribal Population of Orissa*, Bhubaneswar, 1980.

Ota, A.B., (Director SCSTRTI) and S.K. Kar (Director RMRC), *Survey Report on Ecology of Disease Profile of the Tribes of Orissa* with special focus on PTG, Regional Medical Research Centre (RMRC), Bhubaneswar, July, 2007.

Report of the Meriah Agents, Ganjam (1837-1861), Madras, 1855.

Russell, G.E., *Report on Goomsur*, May 11, 1837.

Swain, Saraswati, *Report on the Study of the Health and Morbidity Status of the Tribal Population of Orissa with Special Reference to S.T.D,* (ICMR), New Delhi, October, 1988.

ICMR Bulletin: *Health Status of Primitive Tribes of Orissa*, Vol. 33, No. 10, October, 2003.

Tribal Health, Proceedings of National Symposium, October, 1920, 2006, (RMRC), Bhubaneswar.

Pradhan P., *Socio-Economic Survey Among Penga Kandhas Kashipur Area* (unpublished), Report No. 21, (THRTI), Bhubaneswar, 1971.

Mohanty, P.C., *Handbook on the Kandha of G. Udayagiri* (unpublished), Report No. 48, (THRTI), Bhubaneswar, 1971.

(iii) Records

Chatrapur Revenue Records, John Campbell, Assistant Collectorate to Acting Collector, Nowgam, January, 15, 1839.

Chatrapur Record Room, *Loose correspondence*, J. Campbell to Secretary to Government of India, Berhampur, April 10, 1852, No. 101, 41.

Census of India, 2001.

Orissa Political Records, Vol. 122, E.A. Samuels to Government of Bengal, No. 199, Feb 14, 1856.

Orissa Revenue Records, Vol. 59, Rickets to Government of Bengal, No. 499, March 6, 1837.

(iv) Personal Communication during Fieldwork

Anirudha Dehuri, Jamijhori, Khajuripada Block, Kandhamal District.

Bada Mallik, Rebringia, Baliguda Block, Kandhamal District.

Bholanatha Pradhan, Gatamala, G. Udayagiri Block, Kandhamal District.

Dandapani Kanhar, Kumbabadi, Khajuripada Block, Kandhamal District.

Dirjyo Hikka, Rajanapanasaguda, Laximpur Block, Koraput District.

Raghunath Mallik, Upar Haradabadi, Chikiti Block, Ganjam District.

Raibari Mallik, Lunduriguda, Kukudakhandi Block, Ganjam District.

Sahadev Dehuri, Jhamajhari, Khajuripada Block, Kandhamal District.

Saru Kilo, Disariguda, Khairiput Block, Malkangiri District.

Surendra Mallik, Bhaliaguda, Kukudakhandi Block, Ganjam District.

Taru Pradhan, Jharijhula, Chakapad Block, Kandhamal District.

II. Secondary Sources

(i) Books

Ahmad, M. Lakhrish, *A Village of Kondh*, Cuttack, 1961.

Acharya, P.M., *Odissa Itihasa* (Oriya), Cuttack, 1925.

Akram, Mohammad, *Health Dynamics and Marginalised Communities*, Jaipur, 2007.

Anderson, Clifford R., *Your Guide to Health*, Pune, 1976.

Adak, Dipak Kumar, *et al.*, *Demography and Health Profile of the Tribals,* (ed.), New Delhi, 2003.

Bahadur, K.P., *Caste, Tribes and Culture of India*, Vol. III, New Delhi, 1983.

Balley, F.G., *Tribe, Caste and Nation: A Study in Political Activity and Political Change in High Land Orissa*, Manchester, 1960.

Banarjee, S., *Ethnographic Study of the Kuvi Kondha*, Calcutta, 1969.

Banerjee, R.D., *History of Orissa* (From Earliest Time to the British Period), 2, Vols., Calcutta, 1930.

Basham, A.L., *The Wonder that was India*, New Delhi, 1986.

Basu, B.D., *et al.*, *India Under the British Crown*, London, 1933.

Basu, Sasil, *Tribal Health in India,* Delhi, 1994.

Bhave, V.N., *et al.,* (eds.), *You and Your Health*, New Delhi, 1969.

Boas, N.K., *Cultural Anthropology*, London, 1961.

Boal, B.M., *Kond*, Bhubaneswar, 1984.

Behura, N.K., and K.K. Mohanti, *Tribal Orissa, Reading in Social Anthropology*, New Delhi, 2006.

Behera, Bijay Kumar, *Tribal, Culture, Modernisation and Development- A Study on Kondh Tribe*, New Delhi, 1996.

Basu, Salil, *Tribal Health in India*, Delhi, 1994.

Bryant, J., *Health and Developing World*, London, 1969.

Campbell, George, *Memories of My Indian Career*, London, 1893.

Chakravarty, A.K., *Odisha Itihasa (Oriya),* Cuttack, 1937.

Chakravarty, C., *The Racial History of India*, Calcutta, 1909.

Chaudhuri, Buddhadeb, *Tribal Health; Socio-cultural Dimensions*, New Delhi, 1986.

Chaudhuri, Buddhadeb, *Health, Forest and Development, The Tribal Situation,* New Delhi, 2003.

Cary, S. Pearce, *Dawn on the Kond Hills*, London 1936.

Coupland, R., *The Indian Problems*, London, 1942.

Dalton, E.T., *Tribal History of Eastern India*, Delhi, 1973.

Das, M.N., *Economic and Social Development of Modern India*, Calcutta, 1959.

Douglas, Marry, *Purity and Danger: An Analysis of Concept of Population and Taboo*, London, 1966.

Dash, Bijaylaxmi and Nimal Chandra Dash, *Kondhs an Ethno-botanical Study*, Bhubaneswar, 2009.

Development Hand Book for the Kutia Kandha, Kutia Kandha Development Agency (KKDA,) *Belghar, Phulbani District*, Government of Orissa, Cuttack, 1996.

Das, N.N., *Economic and Social Devlopment of Modern India*, Calcutta, 1959.

Driver, S.C., *The Book of Genesis*, London, 1926.

Elwin, Verrier, *Tribal Myths and Orissa*, London, 1954.

Elwin, Verrier, *The Religion of an Indian Tribe*, London, 1956.

Elwin, Verrier, *The Tribal Art of Middle India*, London, 1951.

Frazer, E.F., *Race and Culture Contacts in Modern World*, New York, 1957.

Friend, Pereira J.E., *Totemism Among Kondhs*, 1904.

Frazer, J.G., *The Golden Bough: A Study in Magic and Religion*, 3rd Edition, London, 1912.

Ghuryl, G.S., *The Scheduled Tribes*, Bombay, 1936.

Gupta, Naveen, *Food and Nutrition, Educational Planning Group*, New Delhi, 1980.

Hiramani, A.B., *Cultural Correlates of Tribal Health*, New Delhi, 1997.

Hayward, V.E.W., (ed.), *The Church as Christian Community*, London, 1966.

Jena, K.C., *Socio-Economic Condition of Orissa during Nineteenth Century*, Delhi, 1978.

Jena, K.C., *Ascendancy of British Raj in Orissa*, Calcutta, 1983.

Jena, Mihir Kumar, Padmini Pathi, Jagganath Dash, Kamala Patnaik and Klaus Seeland, *Forest Tribes of Orissa*, Vol. I, The Dongria Kondh, New Delhi, 2002.

Jena, Mihir Kumar, Padmini Pathi, Jagganath Dash, Kamala Patnaik and Klaus Seeland, *Forest Tribes of Orissa*, Vol. II, Kutia Kondh, New Delhi, 2006.

Jena, B.B., *Orissa People, Culture and Polity*, New Delhi, 1980.

Jain, S.K., *Medicinal Plants*, New Delhi, 1968.

Jain, S.K., *Glimpses of Indian Ethno-botany*, (ed.), Lucknow, 1987.

Jain S.K., *Dictionary of Indian Folk Medicine and Ethnobotany*, New Delhi, 1991.

Jain, S.K., *A Manual of Ethno-botany* (ed.), Lucknow, 1987.

Jose, K. Boban, *Tribal Ethnomedicine Continuity and Change*, New Delhi, 1998.

Kurian, J.C., *Plants that Heal*, Pune, 1995.

Kalla, A.K., and P.C. Joshi, *Tribal Health and Medicine*, New Delhi, 2004.

Knight, J.F., *Family Medicine Care*, Australia, 1982.

Kritiakar, K. R. and Basu, B.D., *Indian Forest Medicinal Plants*, Dehradun, India, 1984.

Keene, H.G., *History of India from the Earliest Times to the Present Day*, London, 1893.

Loudon, J.B., *Social Anthropology and Medicine*, London, 1976.

Mishra, M.K., *Udbhida Sangraha* (Oriya), Berhampur, 2003.

Mohanty, Gopinath, *et al., Cultural Heritage of Ganjam,* Bhubaneswar, 2004.

Mohanty, Gopinath, *et al., Cultural Heritage of Koraput,* Vol. XI Bhubaneswar, 2008.

Mohanty, Gopinath, *et.al., Cultural Heritage of Gajapati,* Bhubaneswar, 2008.

Mohanti, K.K., *et al., Tribes of Koraput*, Koraput, 2006.

Mahatab, H.K., *History of Orissa*, 2, Vols., Cuttack, 1959-60.

Majumdar, B.C., *Orissa in the Making*, Calcutta, 1935.

Mishra P.K., (ed.), *The History and Culture of Indian People*, Vol. IX, Vol. X, Bombay, 1963-65.

Mukharjee, P., *History of Orissa*, Vol. VI, Cuttack, 1964.

Mohanty, Jyotsna, *Tribal Health, Culture and Development in Orissa*, Bhubaneswar, 2004.

Misra, Pramod, *Ecology, Culture and Health, A Primitive Tribe*, New Delhi, 2004.

Mishra, P.K. and J.K. Samal, *Comprehensive History and Culture of Orissa*, Vol. 2, Part 2, New Delhi, 1997.

Mohanty, P.K., *Encyclopedia of Scheduled Tribes of India*, New Delhi, 2006.

Majumdar, D.N., *The Fortunes of Primitive Tribes*, Lucknow, 1944.

Mishra, K., *Koraputra Bivirna Adibasi Jivana* (Oriya), Koraput, 1978.

Moodaliar, A.B.J., *A Legendary Account of the Origin of Konds*, London, 1909.

Mahapatra, Sitakanta, *Modernisation and Ritual: Identify and Change in Santal Society*, Madras, 1986.

Nayak, R.,B.M. Boal and N. Soreng, *The Kondhs: A Hand Book for Development*, New Delhi, 1959.

Nayak, R.K., Boal, B.M. and N. Soreng, *The Kondhs, Indian Social Institute*, Delhi, 1990.

O'Malley, L.S.S., *History of Bengal, Bihar and Orissa under the British Rule,* Calcutta, 1925.

Pattnaik, N., and Patnaik, P.S. Das, *The Kondha of Orissa*, Tribal and Harijan Research-cum-Training Institute (THRIT), Bhubaneswar, 2006.

Patnaik, N.R., *History and Culture of Khond Tribes*, New Delhi, 1992.

Patnaik, N., (ed.), *The Kondh*, (SCSTRTI), Bhubaneswar, 1989.

Paul, K., *Medicine, Magic and Religion*, London, 1925.

Ray, B.C., *Tribes of Orissa*, Bhubaneswar, 1984.

Ray, B.C., *Tribals of Orissa: The Changing Socio-economic Profile*, New Delhi, 1989.

Roy, Kanehan, (ed.), *Education and Health Problems in Tribal Development*, New Delhi, 1989.

Roy, S.C., *Oran Religion and Culture*, New Delhi, 1985.

Russell, R.V. and R.B. Hiralal, *The Tribes and Castes of the Central Provinces of India*, Vol. III, London, 1916.

Satyavati, G.V., A.K. Gupta and N. Tandon, *Medicinal Plants of India*, New Delhi, 1987.

Sharma, Krishan, *The Konds of Orissa*, New Delhi, 1979.

Sharma, A.N., R.K. Gautam, and A.K. Gharami, *Indigenous Health Care and Ethnomedicine*, New-Delhi, 2006.

Sahay, V. S. and P. K. Singh, *Dimensions of Researches in Indian Anthropology*, New Delhi, 2003.

Sahu, L.N., *Hill Tribes of Jeypore*, Cuttack, 1945.

Sahu, L.N., *Jeypore Tribes*, Cuttack, 1942.

Sancheti, K.H., *Best of Health*, Pune, 1994.

Sharma, B.D., *Planning for Tribal Development*, New Delhi, 1984.

Sengupta, Sandhya and Arati Sengupta, *Essentials of Home Science*, Cuttack, 1999.

Swartant, Hubert O., *Your Health and You*, Vol. 2, Lincolnshire, England, 1986.

Samraj, Edison, *Best of Health*, Pune, 1995.

Sengupta, S., *Tree Symbol Worship in India*, Calcutta, 1965.

Thiady, S.B., *Phulbani: The Kondh Land*, Berhampur, 1965.

Thurston, E., *Castes and Tribes of Southern India*, Madras, 1909.

Tribes of Orissa, SCSTRTI, Bhubaneswar, 2004.

Tribhuwan, Robin D., *Medical World of the Tribals*, New Delhi, 1998.

Troisi, J., *Tribal Religion*, New Delhi, 1979.

Tiwari S.K., *Medical Geography Indian Tribes*, New Delhi, 2001.

Tiwari A.N., *Reference Orissa*, New Delhi, 1999.

Troisi, J., *Tribal Religion*, New Delhi, 1979.

Vidyarthi, L.P. and B.K. Rai, *Tribal Culture of India*, New Delhi, 1977.

Winfield, W.W., *A Grammar of the Kui Language, The Asiatic Society of Bengal*, Calcutta, 1928.

(ii) Gazetteers and Manuals

Behuria, N. C., *Orissa District Gazetteer, (Ganjam)*, Bhubaneswar, 1995.

Bell, R.C.C., *District Gazetteer (Koraput),* Cuttack, 1945.

Hunter, W. W., *Imperial Gazetteer of India,* Vol. I, London, 1855.

Maltby, T.J., *Manual of Administration of the Madras Presidency*, Vol. I, Madras, 1885, Vol. III, Madras, 1893.

Maltby, T.J., *The Ganjam District Manual*, Madras, 1918.

O' Malley, L.S.S., *Bengal District Gazetteer (Angul),* Calcutta, 1908.

Senapati, N. and D.C. Kumar, (eds.), *Orissa District Gazetteer (Kalahandi)*, Cuttack, 1966.

Senapati, N. and D.C. Kumar, (eds.) *Orissa District Gazetteer (Boudh-Kondhmal)*, Cuttack, 1983.

(iii) Journals, Proceedings and Reviews

Adivasi.

Calcutta Reviews.

Journals of Orissan History.

Journals of Royal Asiatic Society of Bengal.

Orissa Reviews.

Indian Historical Research Journals.

Indian Historical Reviews.

Indian History Congress Proceedings.

Man in India.

Orissa History Congress Proceedings.

South Indian History Congress Proceedings.

Studies in History and Culture.

Maps and Illustrations

Odisha

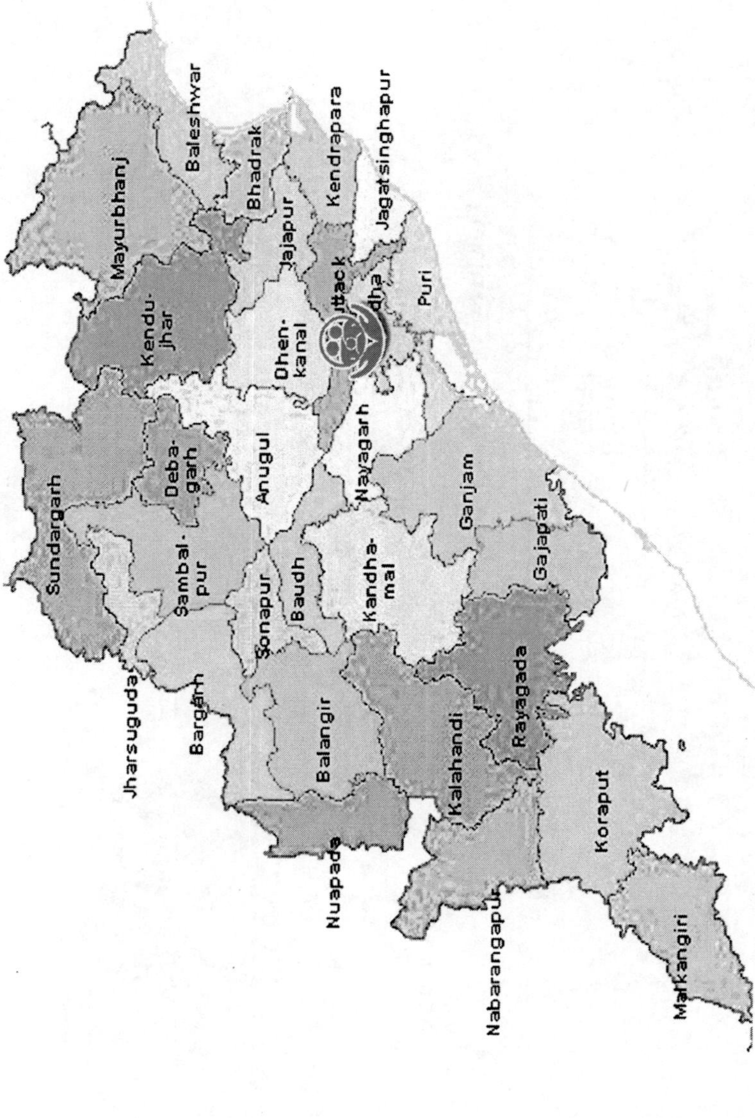
Mayurbhanj
Baleshwar
Bhadrak
Kendrapara
Jagatsinghapur
Jajapur
Kendu-jhar
Dhen-kanal
Puri
Sundargarh
Deba-garh
Anugul
Nayagarh
Ganjam
Sambal-pur
Kandha-mal
Gajapati
Baudh
Sonapur
Jharsuguda
Bargarh
Balangir
Kalahandi
Rayagada
Koraput
Nuapada
Nabarangapur

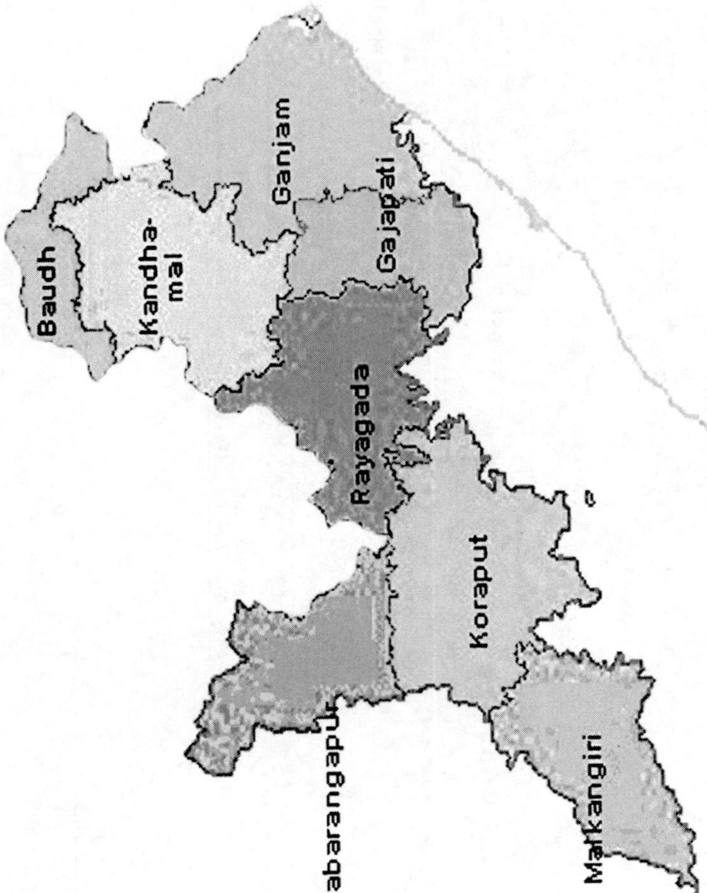

Kondh Inhabited Districts of South Odisha

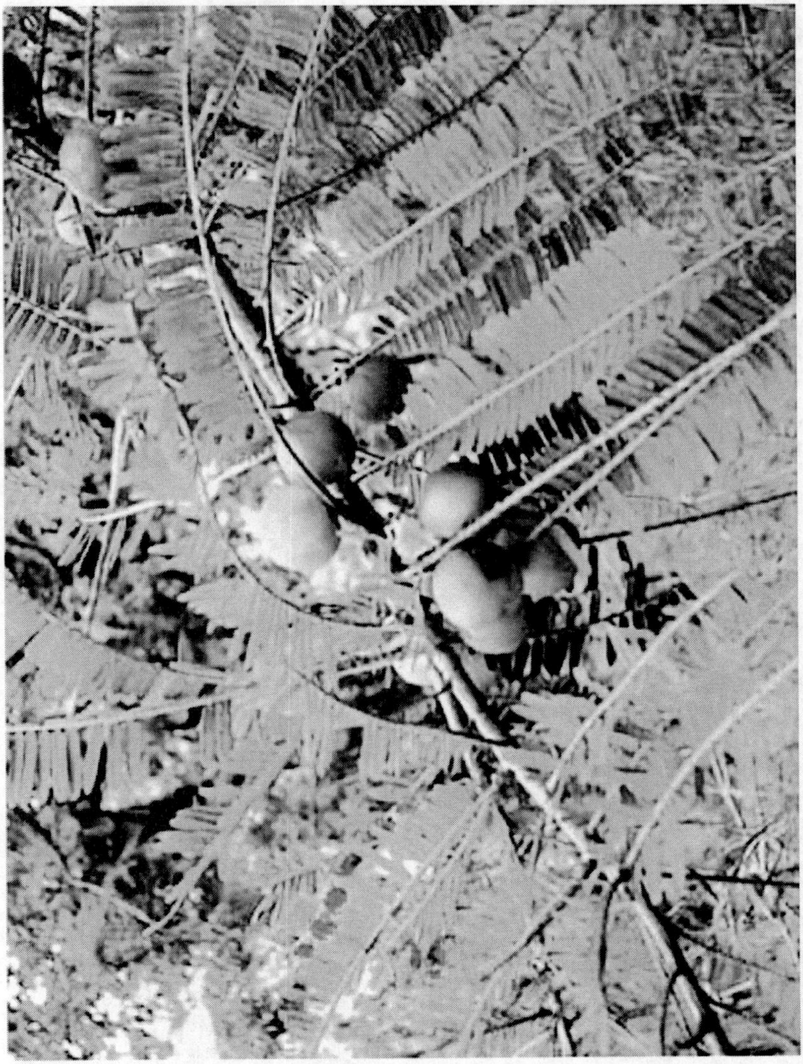

Amla (Phyllanthus Emblica)

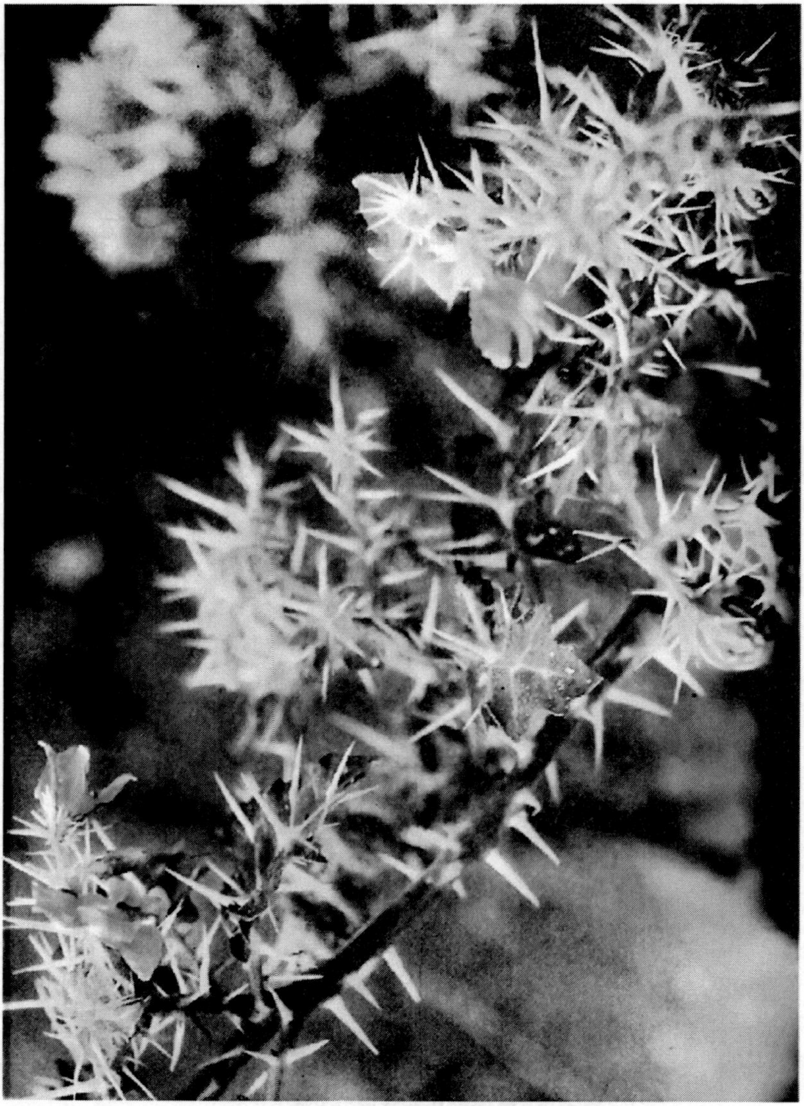

Ankranti (Solanum Xanthocarpum)

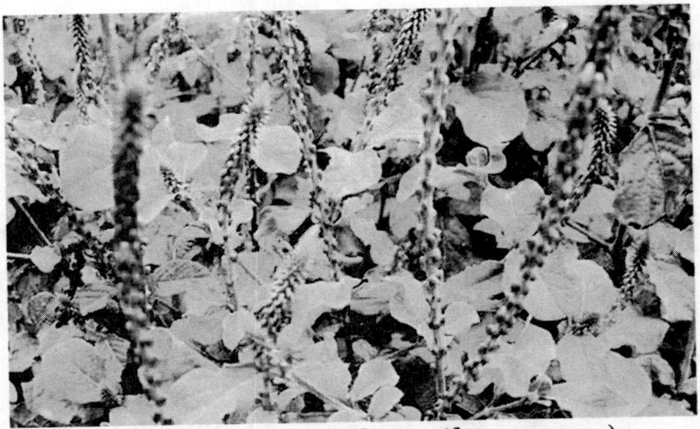

Apamaranga (Achyranthes aspera)

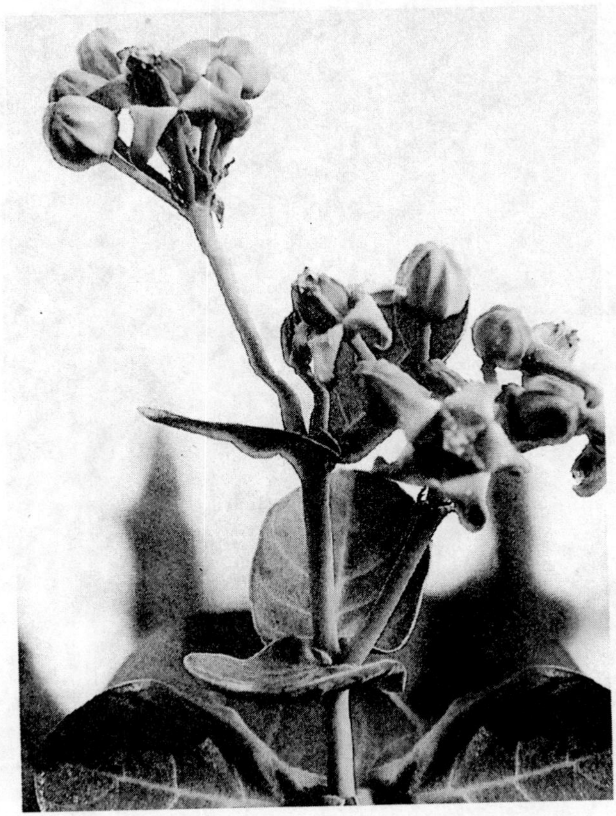

Arakha (Calotropis gigantea)

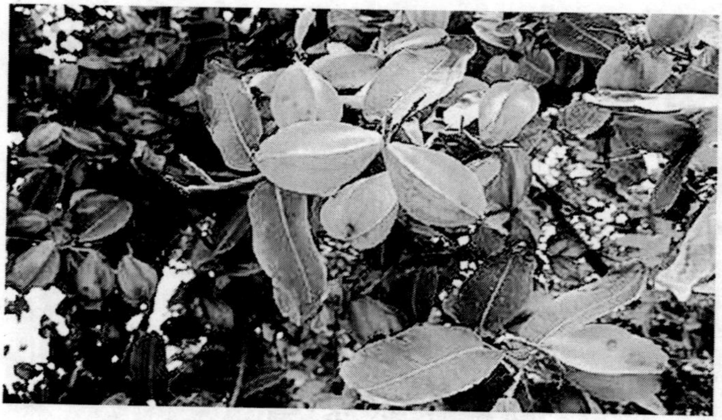

Arjuna (Terminalia arjuna)

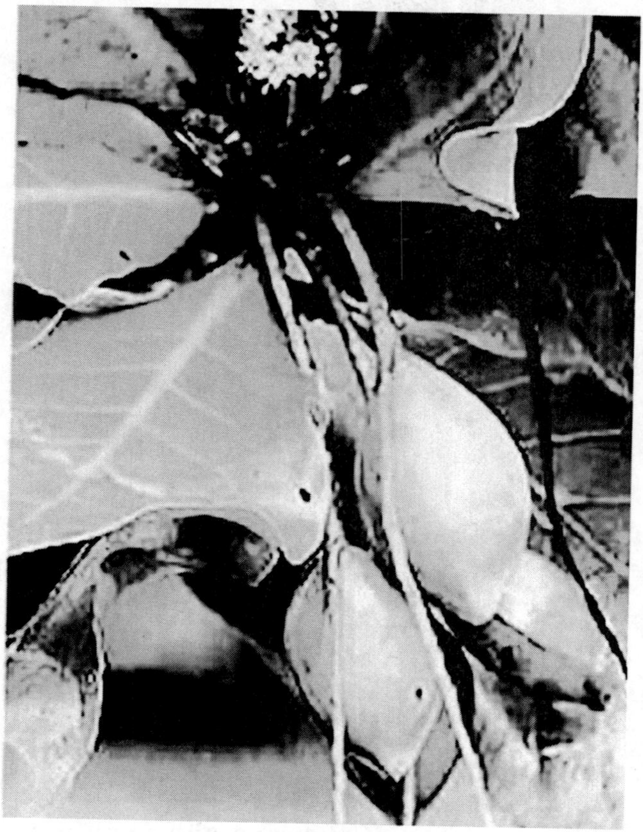

Bahada (Terminalia bellirica)

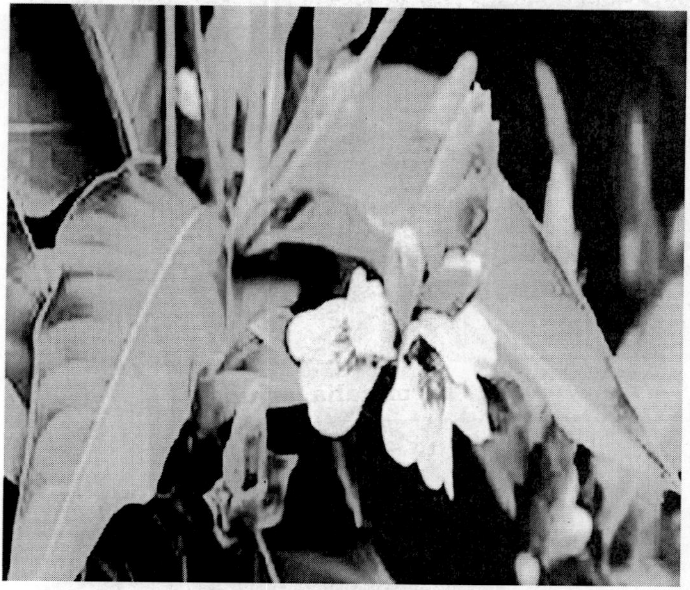

Basanga (Justicia adhatoda)

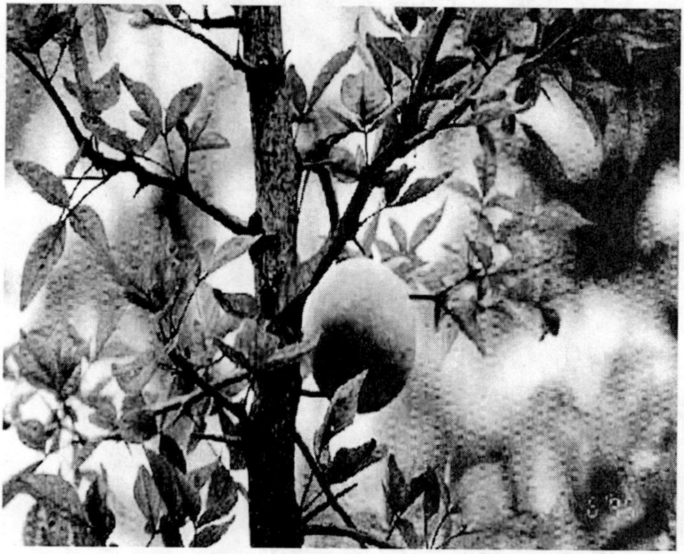

Bela (Aegle marmelos)

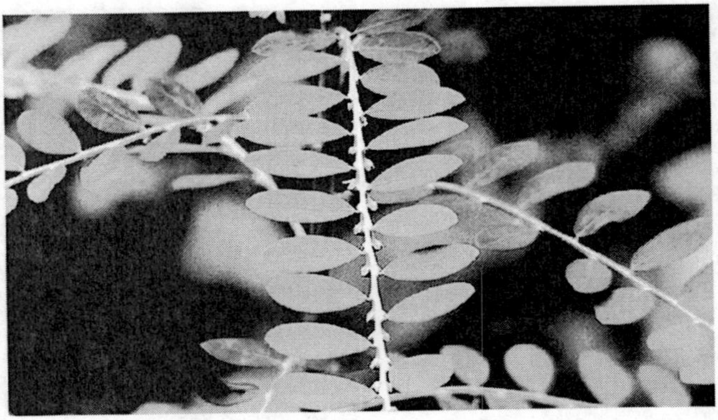

Bhuinamla (Phyllanthus fraternus)

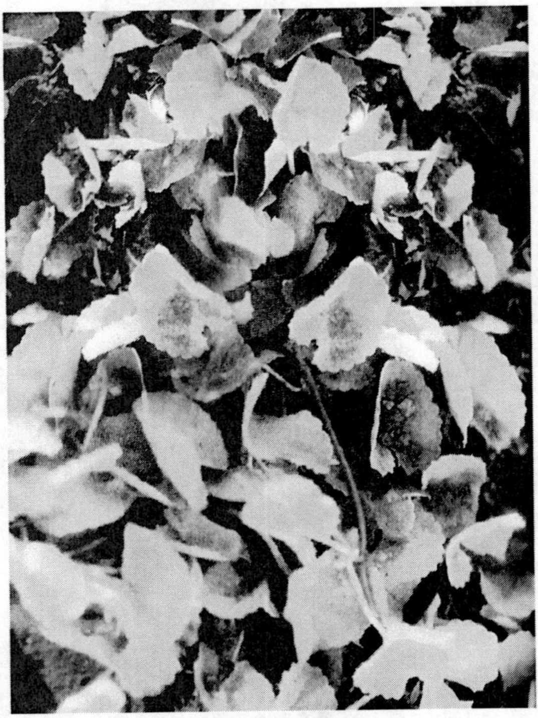

Brahmi (Bacopamonnieri)

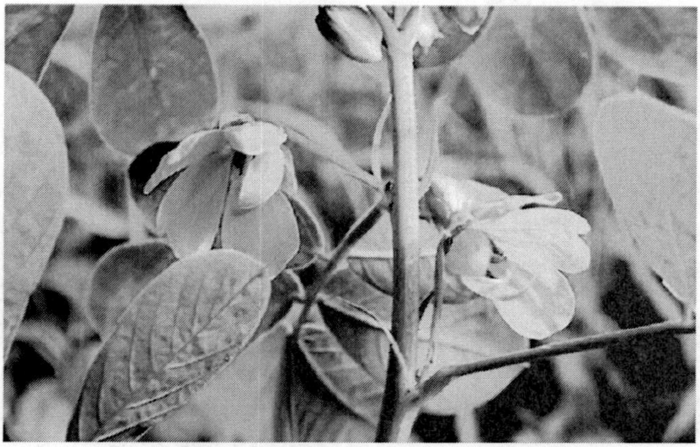

Chakunda (Cassia tora)

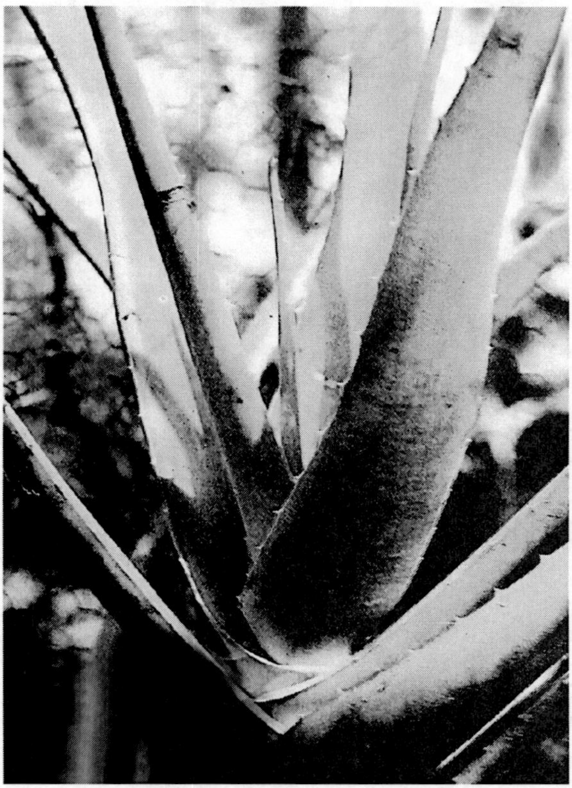

Gheekuanri (Aloe vera)

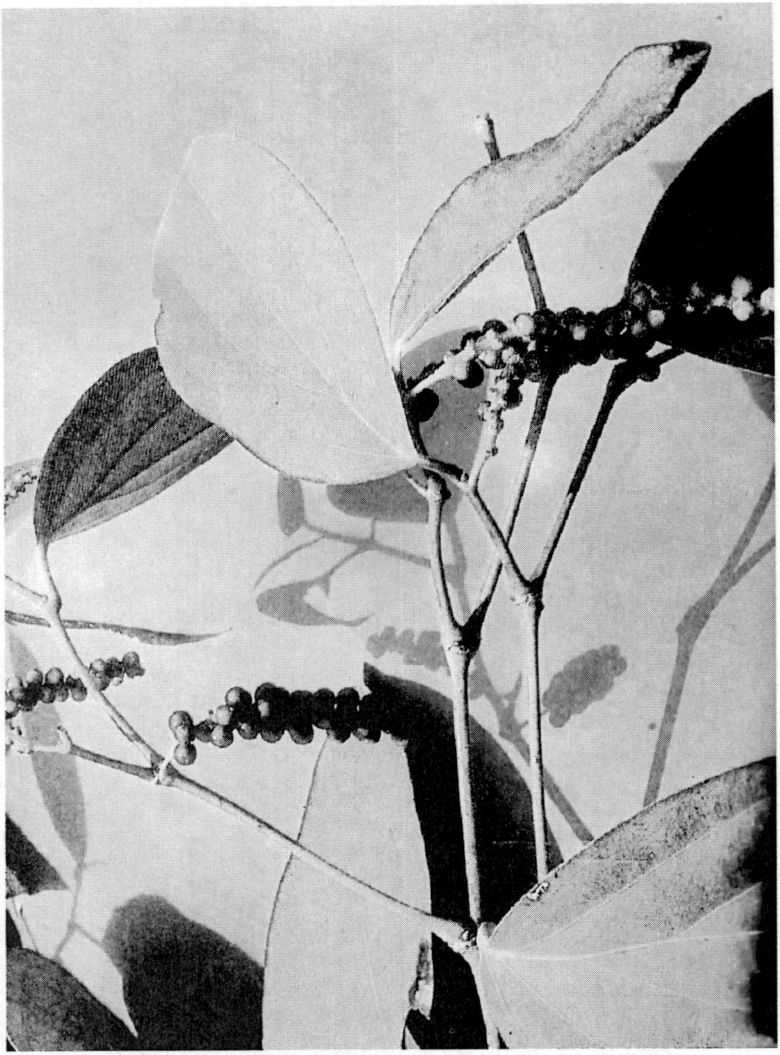

Golamaricha (Piper nigrum)

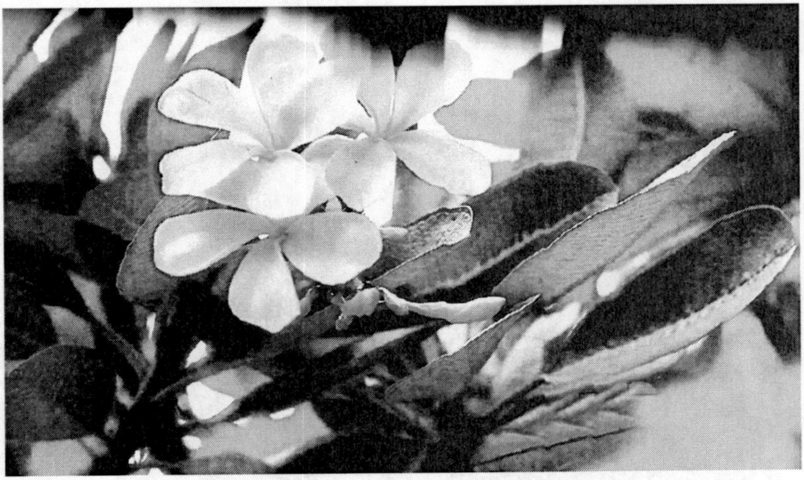

Guluchi (Tinospora cordifolia)

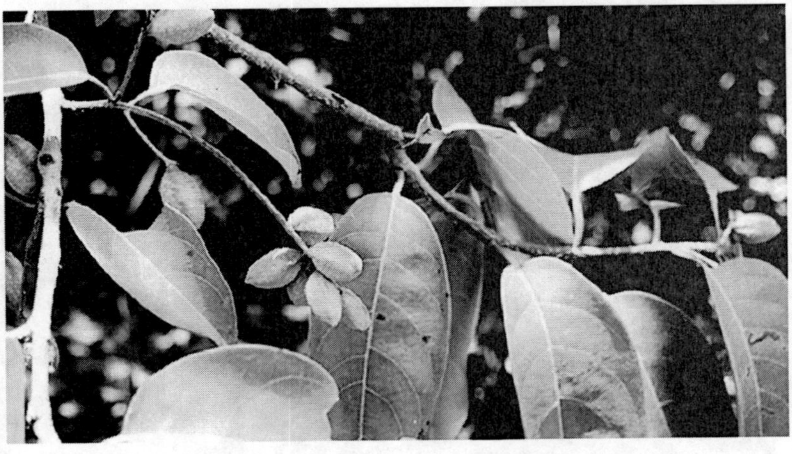

Harida (Terminalia chebula)

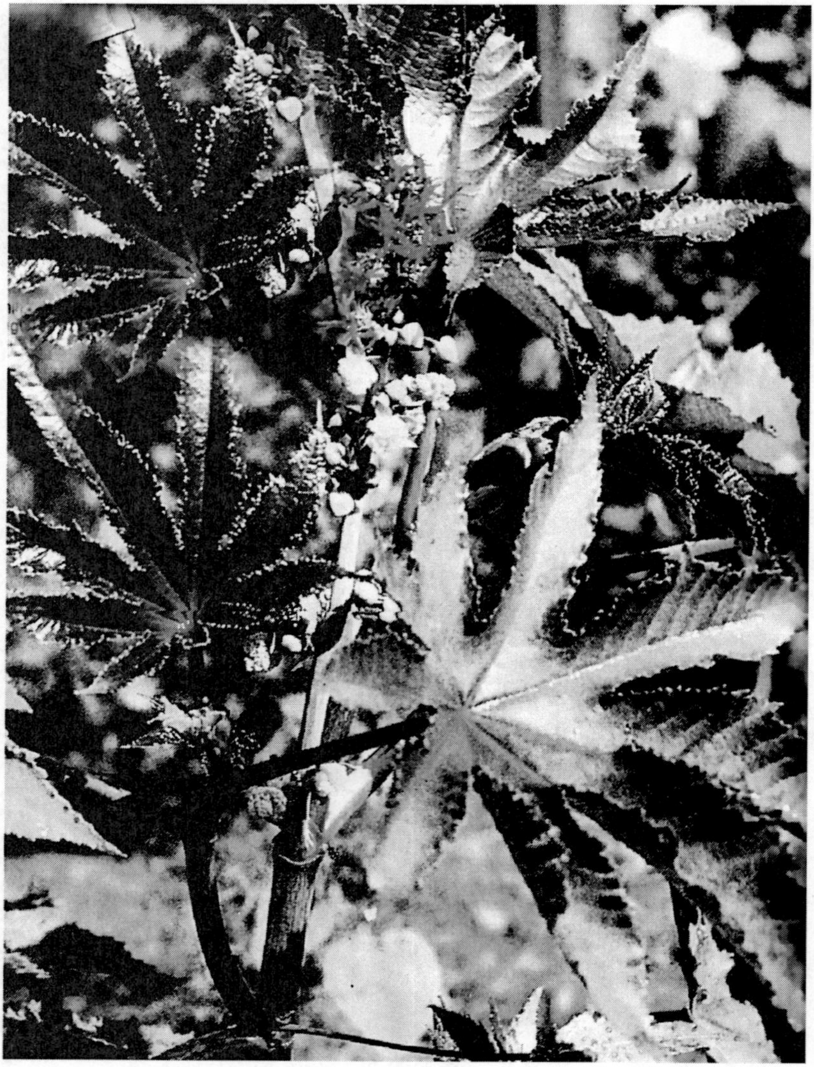

Jada (Ricinus communis)

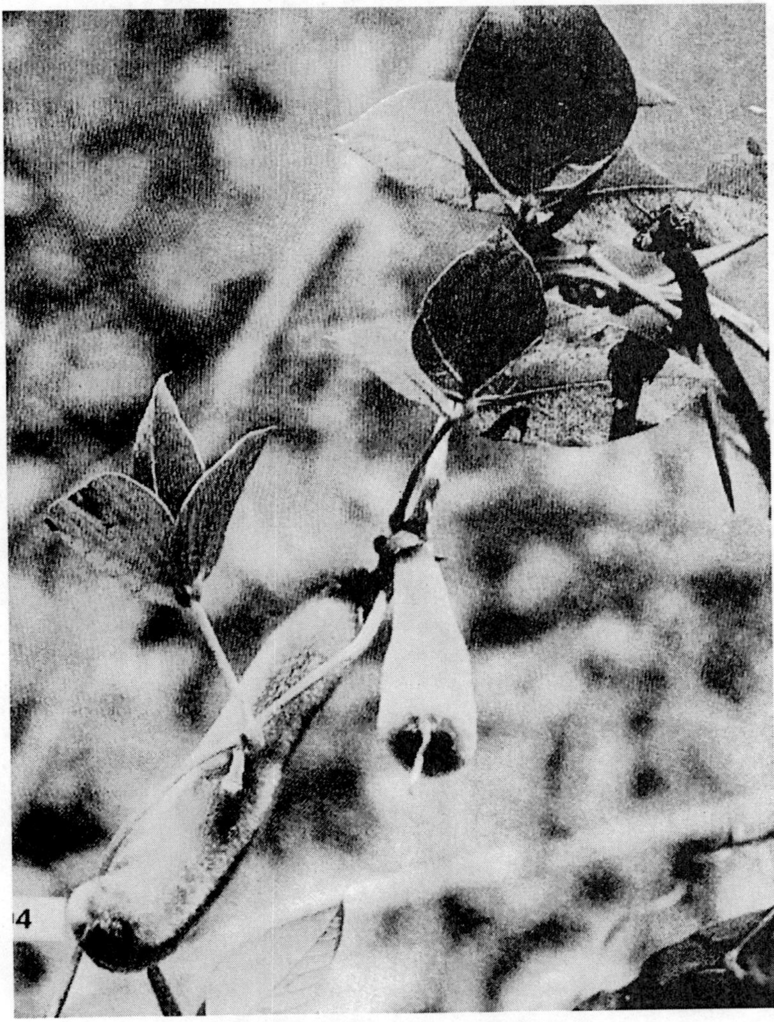

Kaincha (Abrus precatorius)

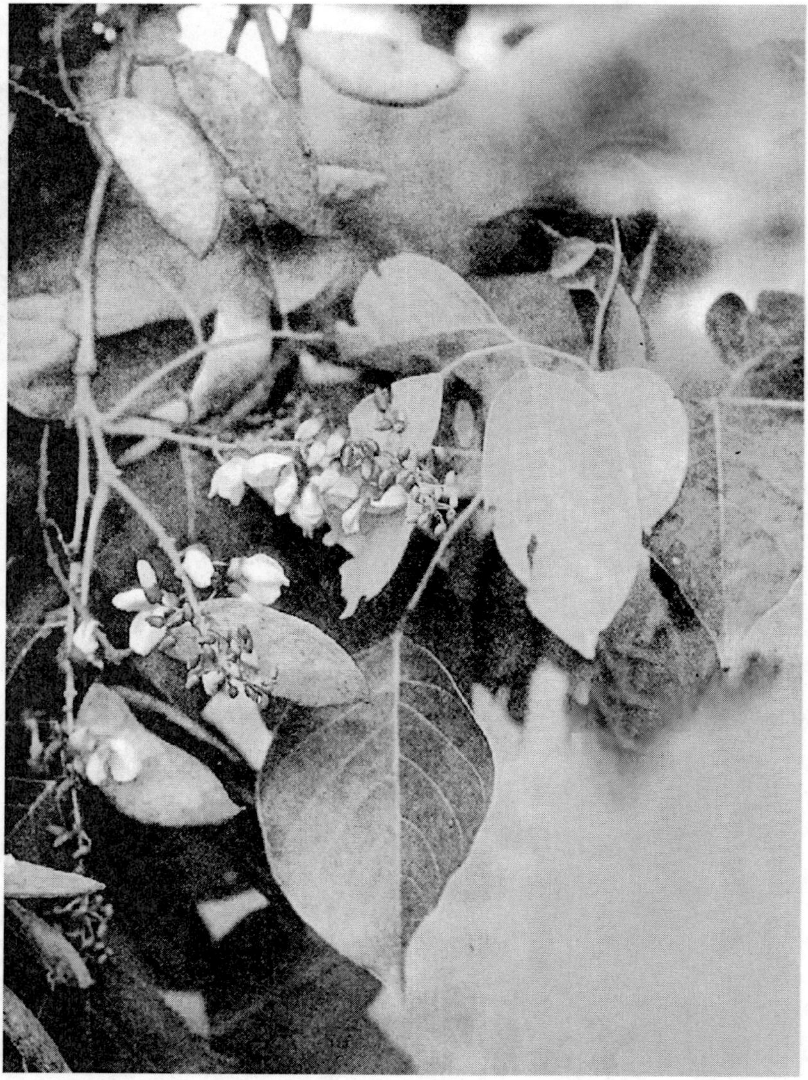

Karanja (Pongamia pinnata)

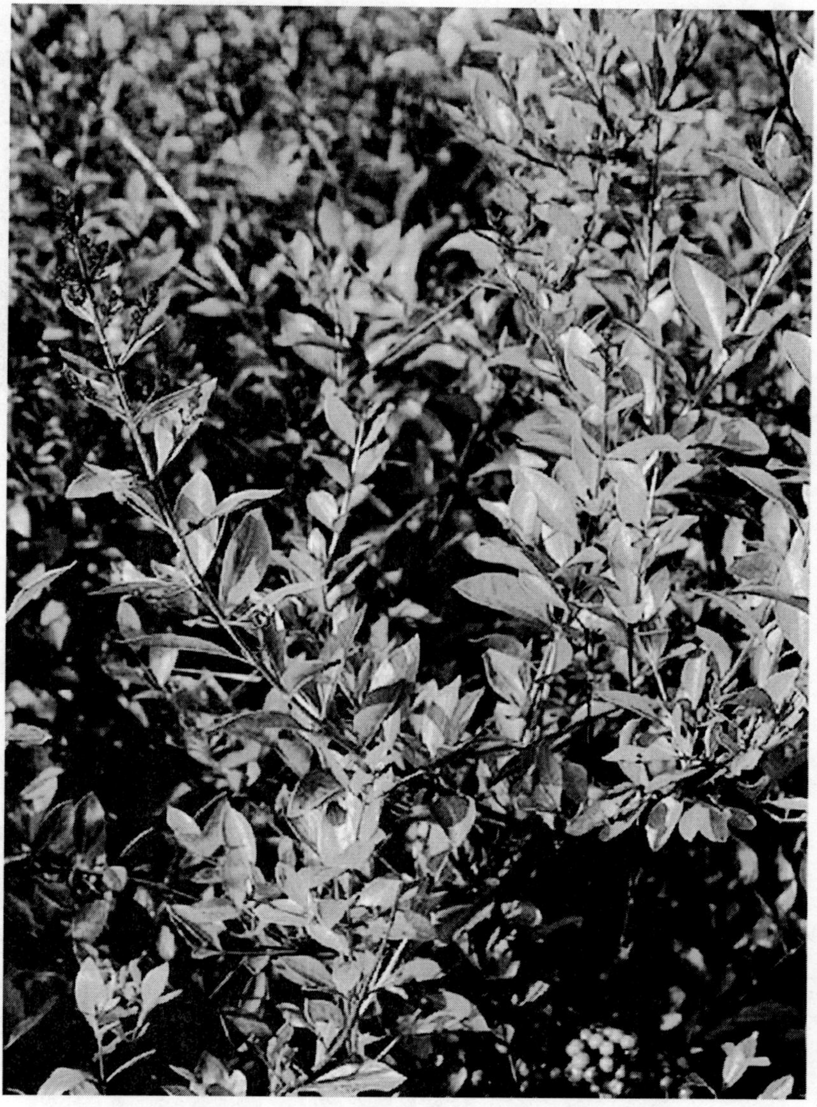

Manjuati (Lawsonia inermis)

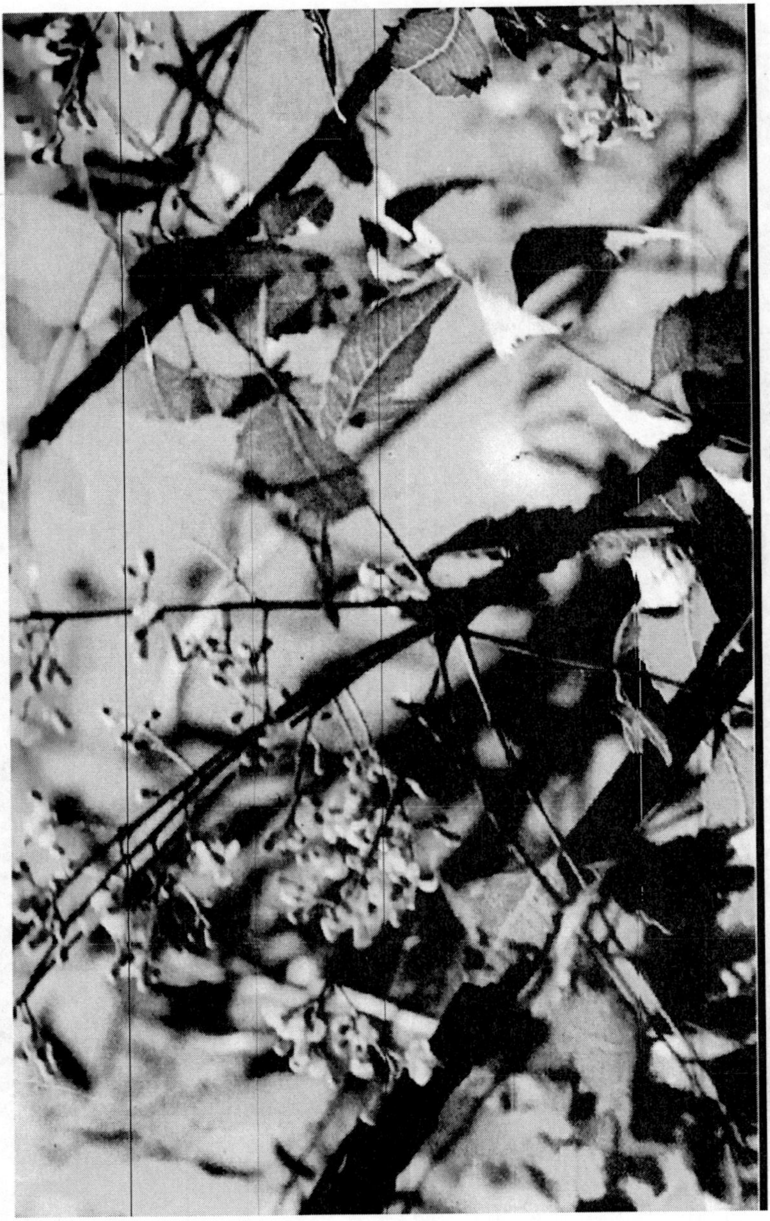

Nimba (Azadirachta indica)

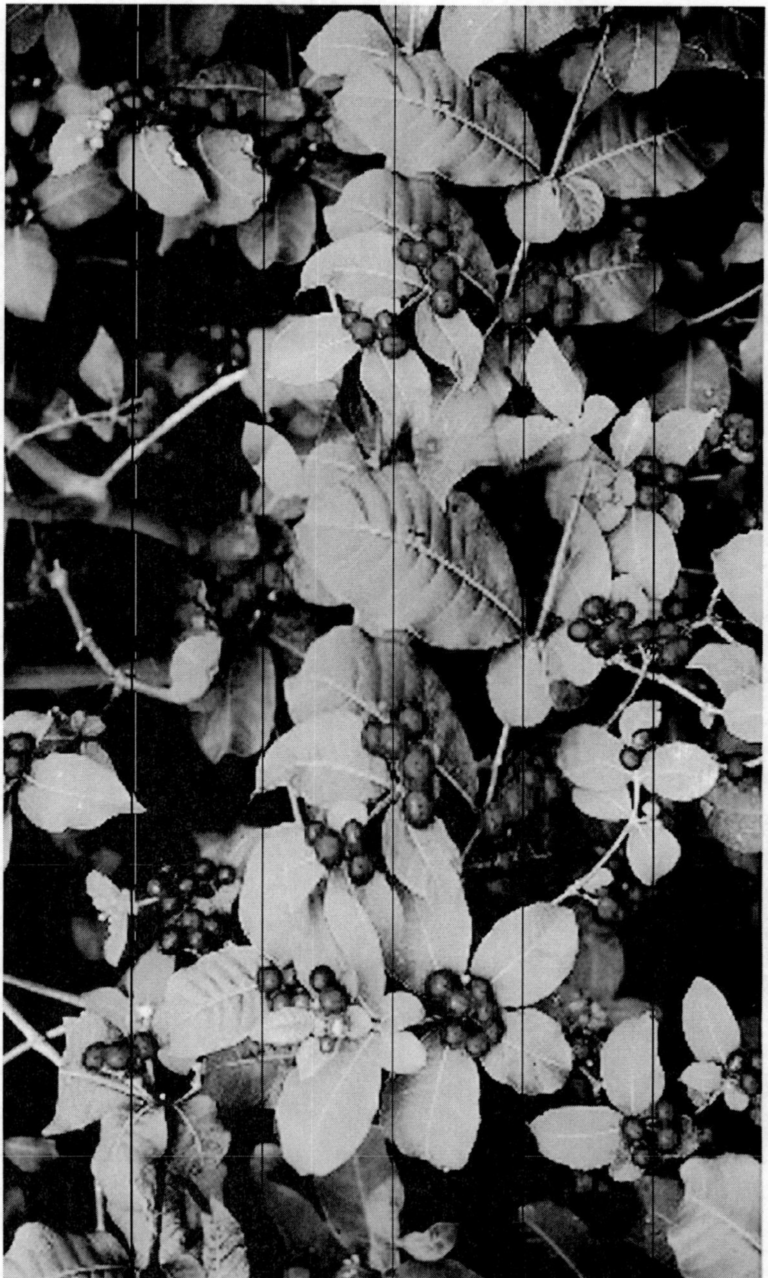

Patalagaruda (Rauvolfia serpentina)

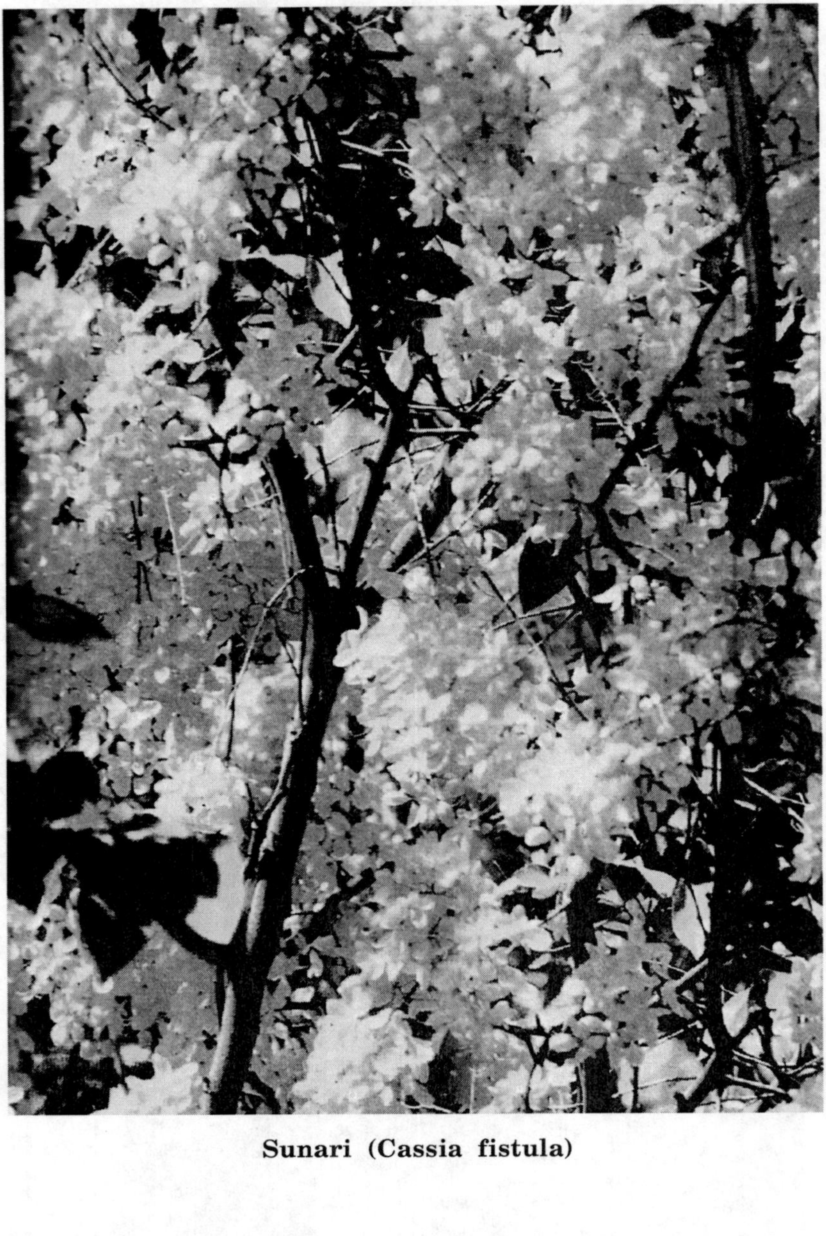

Sunari (Cassia fistula)

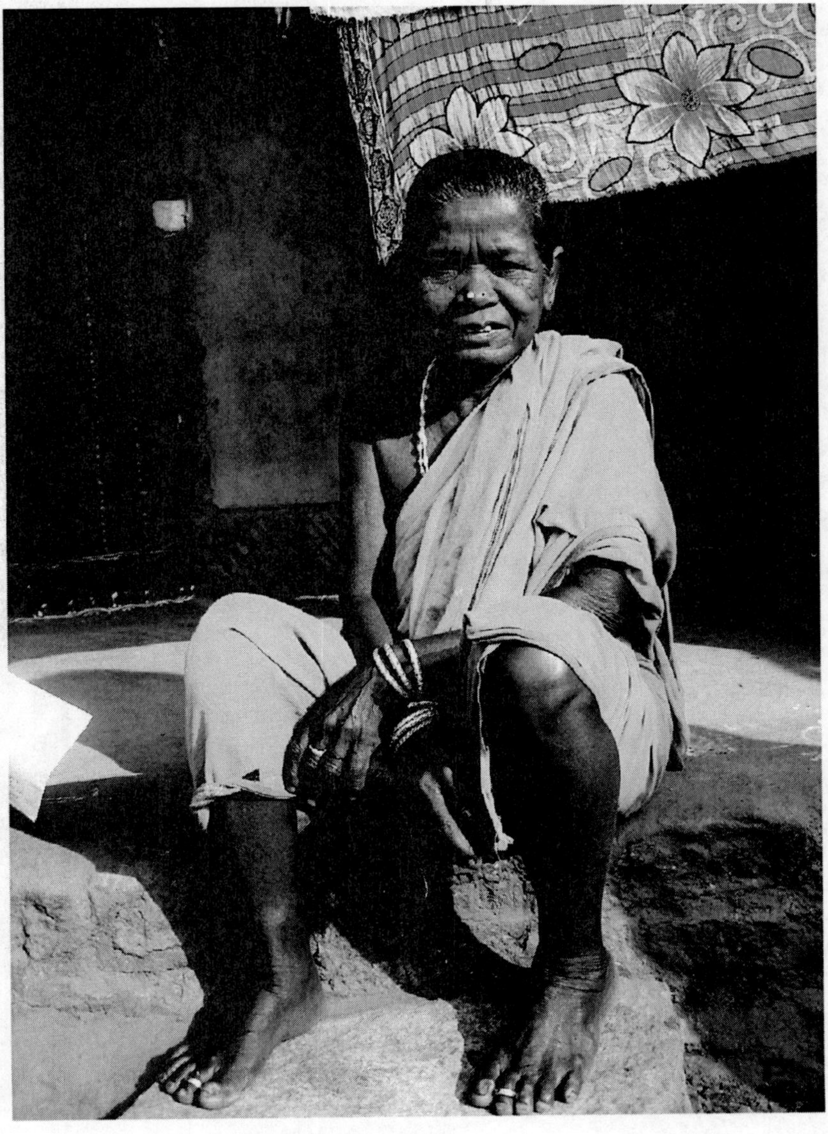

Kondh shamanin

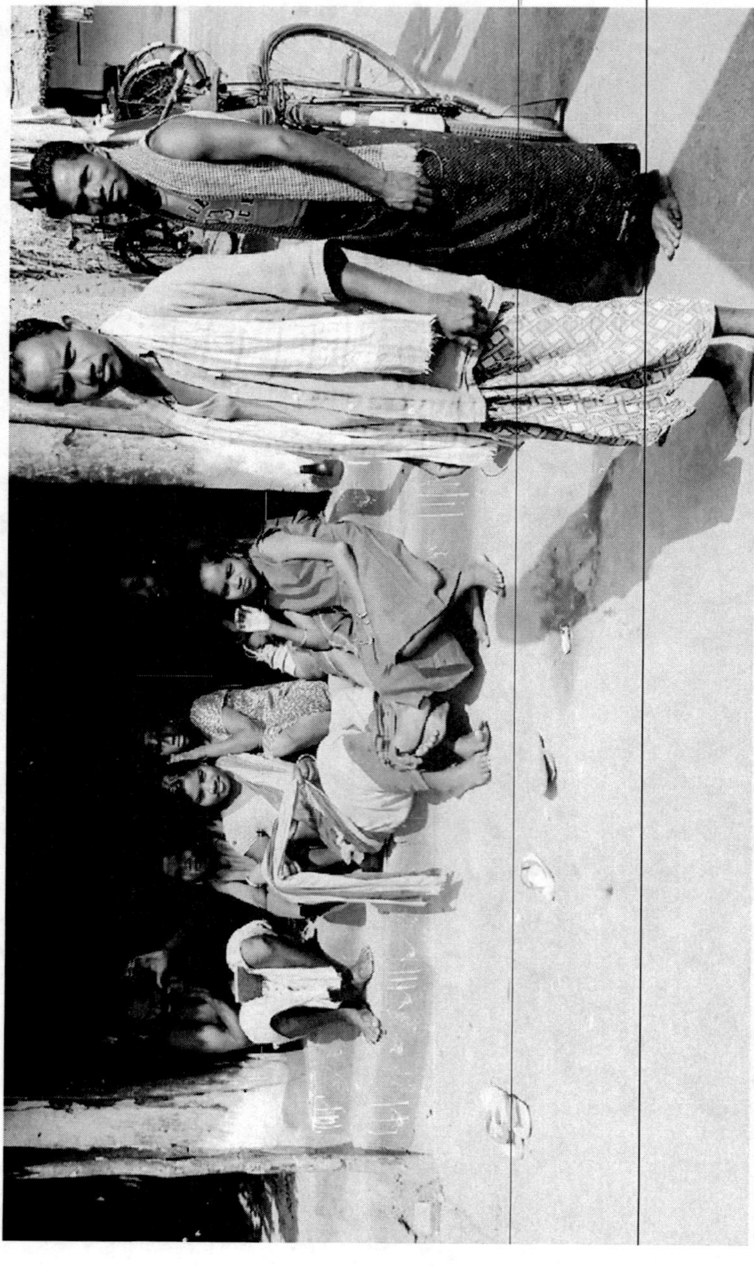

Kondh medicine man with family

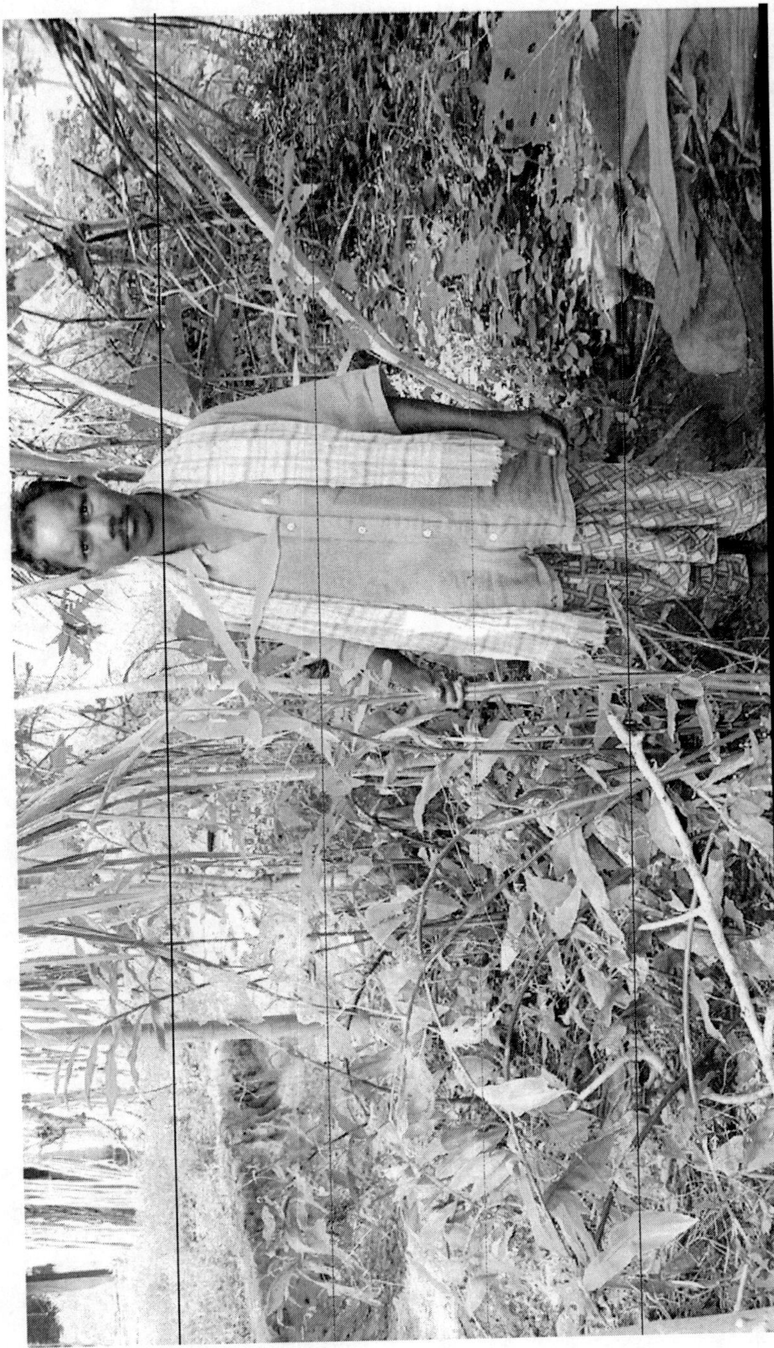

Kondh medicine man carrying Krushna kedar plant

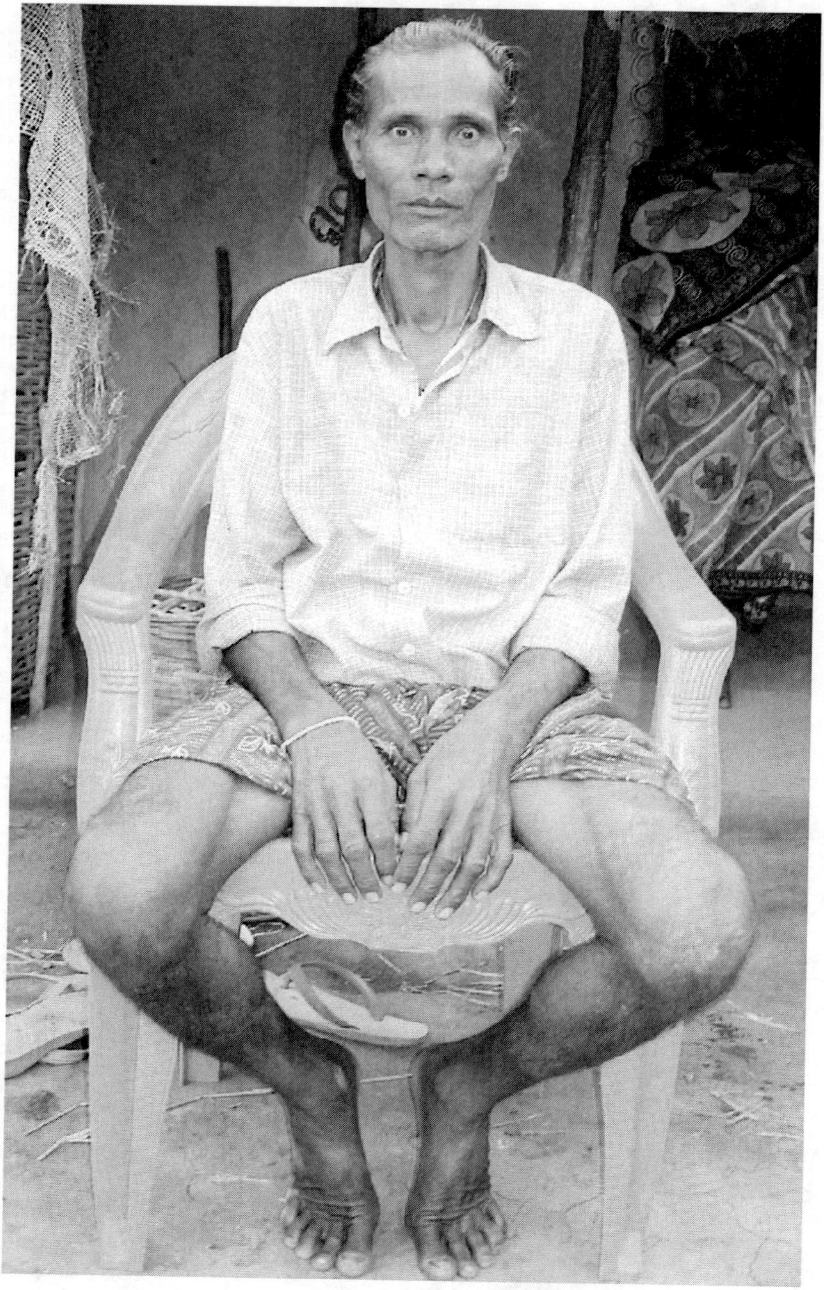

Kondh medicine man

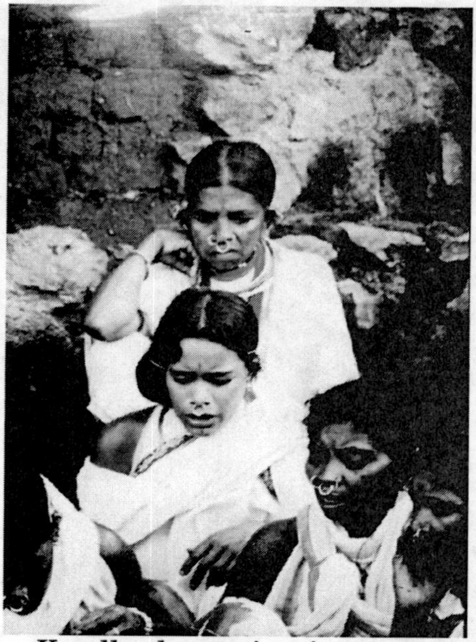

Kondh shamanins in trance

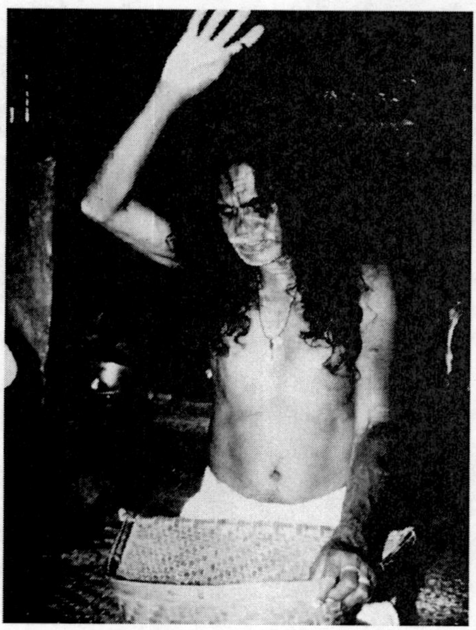

Kondh shaman during healing ritual

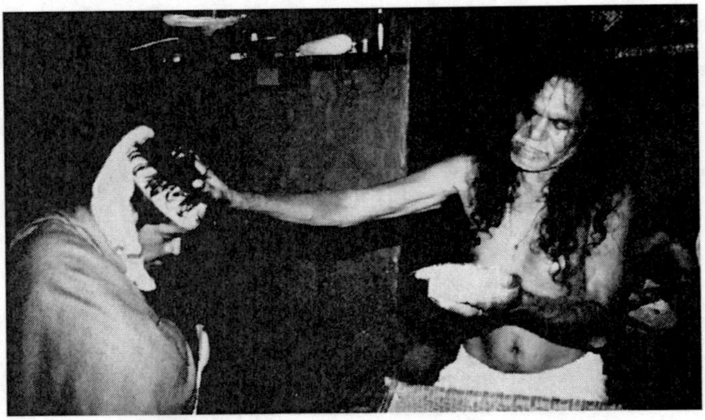

Kondh shaman treating a patient

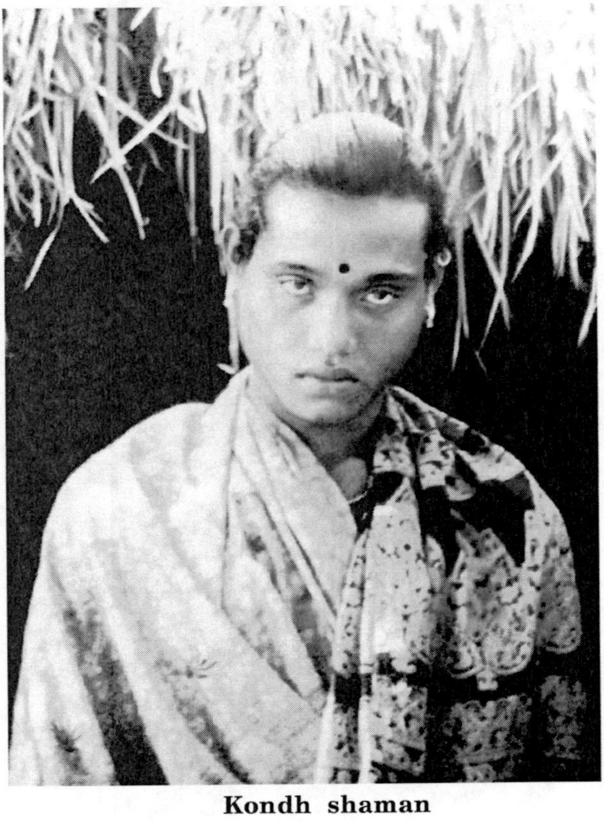

Kondh shaman

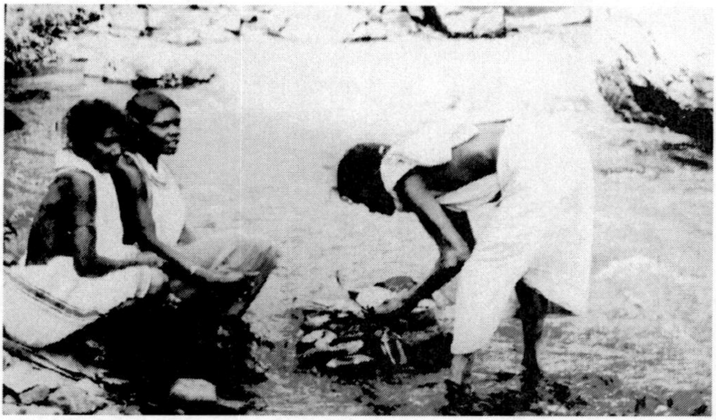

Kondh women performing a ritual in the hill stream

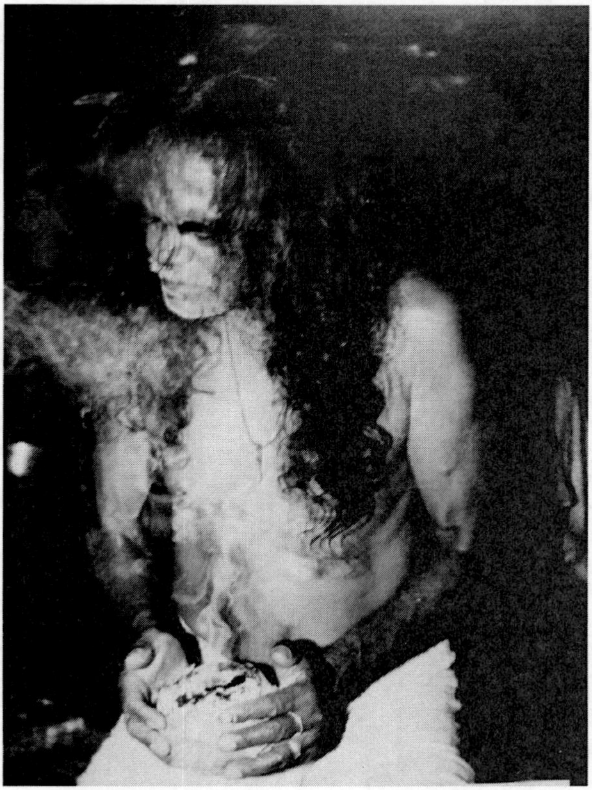

Kondh shaman inhaling smoke of rasin

Index